HEY, DOC!
WHAT'S
WRONG
WITH MY EYE

HEY, DOC! WHAT'S WRONG WITH MY EYE

A GENERAL GUIDE TO EYE SYMPTOMS

JOHN C BARBER, MD, FAAO

Copyright © 2017 by John C Barber, MD, FAAO.

Library of Congress Control Number: 2017909450
ISBN: Hardcover   978-1-5434-2932-9
               Softcover   978-1-5434-2931-2
               eBook   978-1-5434-2930-5

All rights reserved. No part of this book may be reproduced or transmitted in any form or by any means, electronic or mechanical, including photocopying, recording, or by any information storage and retrieval system, without permission in writing from the copyright owner.

Any people depicted in stock imagery provided by Thinkstock are models, and such images are being used for illustrative purposes only. Certain stock imagery © Thinkstock.

Print information available on the last page.

Rev. date: 06/24/2017

To order additional copies of this book, contact:
Xlibris
1-888-795-4274
www.Xlibris.com
Orders@Xlibris.com
762450

To all of my friends and patients who
have asked me about their eyes.

ACKNOWLEDGMENTS

I would like to acknowledge the patience of my wife, Dolores Smith Barber, who has proofread this book and offered comments.

I would also like to thank Albert W Biglan, MD, Thierry Verstraeten, MD, and David J. Kobaly, MD for their comments and encouragement during the writing of this book.

The editors at Tate Publishing have been very helpful and a joy to work with.

The illustrations in the book are licensed by Dreamstime (Dreamstime.com) and are downloaded and used under their license agreement with the author. Figures 1 and 5 were altered by the author through the addition of labels.

CONTENTS

Prologue xi

PART I
Signs and Symptoms

1. Signs versus symptoms 3
2. Red eyes 6
3. Red rimmed eyes 15
4. Itchy burning eyes 21
5. Something in my eye 25
6. Teary eyes, dry eyes 33
7. Lumps and bumps around the eye 38
8. Swelling 42
9. Crossed eyes, wall eyes, and double vision 45
10. Droopy eyelids, ptosis 53
11. Blowout fracture 56
12. Pain 60
13. Flashes and floaters, curtains and shadows 80
14. Rapid vision loss 92
15. Vision color changes 98

PART II
Diseases of All Ages

16. Refractive disorders: myopia, hyperopia, astigmatism and presbyopia 105
17. New ways to correct vision without glasses 121
18. Cataract 130
19. Retinal detachment 166
20. Glaucoma 172
21. Corneal transplants 193
22. Age-related macular degeneration 211
23. Uveitis 219
24. Acquired (adult) strabismus or muscle palsy 226
25. Diabetes and the eye 232
26. Thyroid eye disease 240
27. AIDS, Acquired Immunodeficiency Syndrome 245

PART III
Eye Problems of Children

28. Embryology and congenital eye problems 251
29. Lacrimal (tearing) problems in children 255
30. Other congenital eye defects 258
31. Acquired eye problems in children 273
32. Pink eye or conjunctivitis 293
33. Hereditary diseases in children 298

PROLOGUE

Rationale for this book

"Hi Doc, I'm glad I ran into you. I've been having a problem with my eye. Can you look at it and tell me what to do?"

This is a question I am asked with increasing frequency, now that I have retired from my practice of ophthalmology. This happens at cocktail parties, grocery stores, the opera, my church and any place I might run into a friend or former patient.

This custom used to irritate me when I viewed these questions in social settings as a way to avoid making an appointment with a doctor and paying them (or me) for the evaluation and advice.

Now that I am not practicing, I look at these questions as an opportunity to educate people and be sure that they are referred to a general ophthalmologist or the right subspecialist, saving them a step in the process.

Many primary care physicians admit to major gaps in their knowledge of eye diseases and are uncomfortable in diagnosing and treating eye problems. Most medical schools do not want to devote the time on specialties to teach them adequately, even for general practitioners. Knowing what is explained in this book may help you in seeking needed care from the appropriate eye care provider. The information in this book should allow you to ask appropriate questions and better understand the answers that are given.

Throughout my practice years, I prided myself in being able to explain diseases to the patient, to put the problem in common terms that the patient can understand, and to use understandable metaphors to explain what is wrong and how to fix it. I believe that the more people know about their diseases, the better they can follow the needed therapy and make better decisions when choices are presented to them.

In this book I will explain what common symptoms mean and when they indicate a serious problem, or an emergency, and when signs and symptoms can be ignored. The first section of the book concerns the signs and symptoms of common eye problems.

The later chapters will explain the common eye problems like cataracts, retinal detachments, glaucoma and age-related macular degeneration and how they are treated. Diseases like macular degeneration, thyroid eye disease, diabetic eye problems, and crossed eyes will be explained. I will also explain what is involved in the treatment and surgical procedures along with the major complications that occur during and after medical and surgical therapies. I have included a section about childhood diseases and there is a separate chapter on AIDS problems and treatments.

I spent almost my entire career in medical institutions, either being taught or teaching others. I graduated from Washington University Medical School in St. Louis and completed a rotating internship at St. Luke's Presbyterian Hospital, also in St. Louis.

After two years at the U.S. Food and Drug Administration I went on to a Residency in Ophthalmology at the Medical College of Virginia in Richmond. I was attracted to academic medicine and a specialty in diseases of the front part of the eye so I spent two years under the tutelage of Dr. Claes H. Dohlman at The Massachusetts Eye and Ear Infirmary in Boston, a part of Harvard Medical School.

My first faculty position was in 1973 at the University of Texas Medical Branch in Galveston (UTMB), teaching residents and students and seeing private and clinic patents. I became chairman of the department in 1981. UTMB was the state hospital for Texas so we saw patients from all over the state. They were sent to us and we could not send them on so we had to do everything in ophthalmology for these people. I saw many interesting cases from all walks of life. There were twelve residents in the clinic and each faculty member had a private practice in their specialty.

During the recession of the 1980's our clinic was very busy.

In 1991 I left Galveston, for personal reasons, to run the ophthalmology residency program at St. Francis Medical Center in Pittsburgh. Supervising six residents caused me to see many patients with a wide variety of diseases. We worked closely with residencies in radiology, psychiatry, rehabilitation, internal medicine, oral-maxillofacial surgery. I also had a part-time referral practice for diseases of the front half of the eye.

Throughout my practice I prided myself in being able to explain situations and diseases to my patients and answer their questions in language they could understand. I have tried to avoid technical language and medical jargon where possible and explain it when it occurred.

Eye anatomy and physiology

The eyes and the tissues around them are very complex and are often poorly understood by many people, even doctors who are not specialized in eye care. Much of the medical terminology in ophthalmology, which has evolved over many years, is based on the Greek language rather than Latin. Terms describing the conditions involving the eye are often different from those used for similar conditions in other organs. All of this leads to a specialized language for ophthalmology which is often very different from the rest of medicine.

When I taught in medical school, I had a multiple choice question on the examination for the student to choose the correct spelling of the word ophthalmology. I could always tell when the students reached that question, because they always flipped back to the first page to look for the spelling in the title for the exam. I was always careful to title the exam "The Eye Exam." A significant number got it wrong every time.

There are so many specialized tissues in the eye and the surrounding structures that a large variety of diseases can affect the eyes and the adjacent parts of the face. Many common diseases such as high blood pressure and diabetes can be diagnosed by examining the eyes.

In order to understand the eye and the things that can go wrong with it, it is necessary to know the names of the parts and how they function, so I will try to give the reader a crash course in ophthalmology.

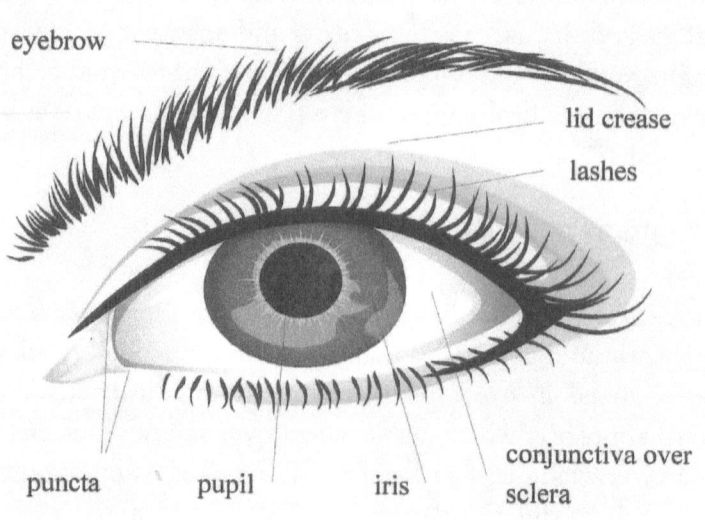

Starting from the front of the eye we first see the eyelids. The upper eyelid moves a lot, but the lower eyelid does not appear to move. Blinking is a normal function which spreads the tears across the front of the eye, keeping it moist. Lid action also wipes away superficial foreign bodies like dust and pollen. Closing the eyelids wipes tears toward the nasal side and pumps them down the tiny ducts that go from the eyelids, through the eye socket and nasal bones, and into the nose. That is why the nose runs when we cry.

Thyroid disease affects the number of times a minute that the eyelids blink. If blinking slows down, the tears dry up and the eyes become uncomfortable. Reading or staring at close work, such as sewing, will slow the blinking rate, making the eyes feel tired or dry after several minutes.

For various reasons the upper eyelid may droop. The term for this is ptosis, with a silent "P." (toe sis). The patient looks sleepy or appears to be winking at someone. To see out from under the drooping eyelid, the patient often tilts their head back to look down and peek out under the drooping eyelid.

The lower eyelid may become lax with age, or chronic allergic swelling, making it a bag of tissue. Occasionally the bag becomes so heavy, or the eyelid so stretched, that the eyelid pulls away from the eye. This is called lagophthalmos. Usually there is a pool of tears along the edge of the lower eyelid where it rests against the eyeball. When the lid sags, these tears drop down into the conjunctiva behind the eyelid. From there the upper eyelid cannot pick up the tears to spread them over the eye to keep it moist.

The eye is dry, but the tears run out over the lax eyelid and run down the cheek creating a paradox of tearing from a dry, irritated eye.

When there is nerve or muscle damage to the upper eyelid, it may droop and close the eye partially or totally, creating ptosis.

Some children are born with this and it may be genetic and run in families. It can also be caused by tumors, stroke, diabetes and high blood pressure and other diseases in adults.

The eyelids contain a plate of cartilage, the tarsal plate, which stiffens the areas near the edges. This prevents curling of the edges and maintains contact between the lid and the eyeball. Certain diseases, like trachoma and pemphigoid, and trauma, can cause deformity of these plates, interfering with eyelid functions.

Eye lashes are the protective hairs that line the edges of the eyelids; they catch foreign bodies like dust, dandruff and lint and keep them out of the eye. They should point away from the eye, but when they are misdirected, they may cause problems.

Occasionally they may grow in the wrong direction, rubbing or scratching the eye. This also happens with scarring diseases, like pemphigoid, and must be treated for the comfort of the patient.

Several diseases cause some of the lashes to turn prematurely grey and fall out, a condition called madarosis. One of the common glaucoma drugs, LumiganR (bimatoprost), makes lashes darker and thicker. It is now available from your plastic surgeon as LatisseR to use to darken eye lashes cosmetically.

Children are often born with eyelid problems which I will address later. See Children's eye problems.

The back of the eyelids and the white part of the front of the eyeball are covered by a thin, clear tissue called conjunctiva. It reflects back upon itself from the back of the eyelids to the front of the eyeball forming a sac above, below, and toward the temple.

Conjunctiva lines the eyelids and front of the eyeball and walls off the eyelid opening into the body. The reflection of the conjunctiva from the eyelids to the eyeball also keeps contact lenses from going back behind the eye when they come off of the cornea.

There are blood vessels in the conjunctiva so that it appears pink and becomes red when it is irritated causing these vessels to dilate. Certain things can collect in the tissue of the conjunctiva causing it to change color, such as silver (argyria), bile pigments (jaundice), skin pigments, and blood (hemoglobin staining), to name a few. The conjunctiva is full of white blood cells, antibodies, and enzymes that protect the body from harmful bacteria and toxic chemicals.

The Lacrimal Apparatus

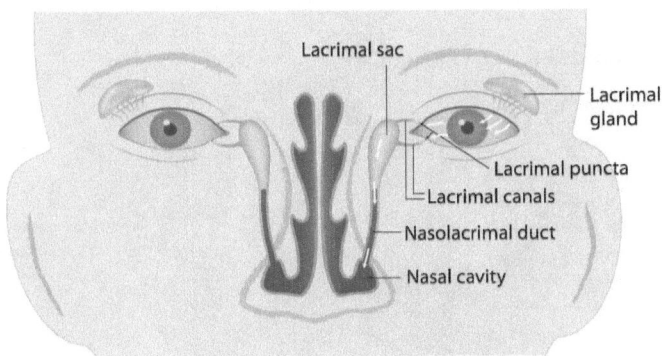

During development of the face, the glands that make tears and saliva are differentiated from embryonic tissue. There is a large lacrimal gland that is situated in the upper, outer quadrant of each eye socket. It develops ducts that go through the upper cul-de-sac of the conjunctiva to discharge tears on the surface of the eye under the upper eyelid. Several similar glands are clustered around the jaw and discharge saliva into the mouth through ducts from each gland. The mesoderm differentiates into hundreds of small lacrimal glands that are spread throughout the conjunctiva.

These secrete tears directly onto the conjunctival surface.

Tears drain from the eye through tiny ducts at the nasal ends of the upper and lower eyelids. These ducts are called canaliculi.

The upper and lower ducts from each eye join to form a common canaliculus that drains into a lacrimal sac near the nose. This sac drains through a tube (nasolacrimal duct) that discharges into the nasal passage where the tears are absorbed. This is why the nose runs during crying.

JOHN C BARBER, MD, FAAO

The Anatomy of the Eye

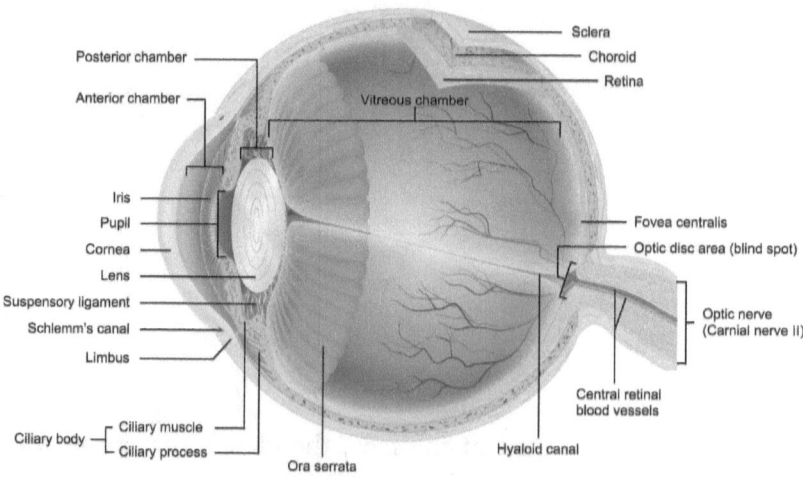

There is a round, clear window in the front of the eye, called the cornea. The surface of the cornea is covered by a thin tissue called epithelium which is similar to conjunctiva, but without any blood vessels or mucin producing cells, called goblet cells.

The cornea, itself, does not contain blood vessels. This absence of blood vessels delays healing and makes the cornea susceptible to enzymatic dissolution. The cornea has an affinity for water which makes it swell and become cloudy. There is an active system in the back lining of the cornea, the endothelium, which constantly pumps excess water from the cornea, keeping it clear. Failure of that system allows the cornea to swell and become cloudy, decreasing vision. The absence of blood vessels creates a prime location to transplant donor tissue into from unrelated persons.

The first corneal transplant, done in 1904, was one of the first successful tissue transplants, because of this favored recipient site.

The cornea is the optical surface of the eye. The curvature of the cornea begins the process of focusing the light within the eye to create the image on the retina, which is the film in the camera.

If the cornea is too flat, the eye is farsighted. If it is too curved, the eye is nearsighted. Irregularities, warping, or scarring of the cornea may distort the visual image.

The round, colored part of the eye which is plainly visible is called the iris. It is inside of the eye, behind the cornea, in a space filled with fluid called the anterior chamber. The iris is pigmented and gives the color to the eye. It is made up of lacy fibers, muscles, nerves, and blood vessels. There is a thick layer of pigment which covers the back surface, blocking light from entering the eye. The center of the iris has a round hole that allows light to enter the eye. This hole, the pupil, can be enlarged (mydriasis) or constricted (miosis) by the muscles in the iris, thus regulating the amount of light that enters the eye. The pupil constricts with bright light and when looking a nearby objects and dilates in darkness and when looking at distance. Some diseases, such as Horner's syndrome (a sympathetic innervation problem) and neuro-syphilis, interfere with these reactions.

The space filled with fluid, between the cornea and iris, is called the anterior chamber. The watery fluid, called aqueous humor, is secreted within the eye, behind the iris, in the posterior chamber.

It flows around the lens in the eye and through the pupil into the anterior chamber. This fluid bathes the lens and the back surface of the cornea and brings nutrition to both. The fluid leaves the eye through a filter or meshwork, called the trabecular meshwork, located where the base of the iris meets the edge of the cornea or front end of the sclera. If this mesh collapses, restricting the flow of the aqueous humor from the eye, the pressure in the eye will increase and cause damage. This is called glaucoma. The rise in pressure is similar to partially covering the end of a water hose with your thumb to make it squirt farther.

Behind the pupil is a clear flattened ball which is the lens. It adds to the focusing of light onto the retina to allow sharp vision.

It is made of layers of clear tissue surrounded by a thin, clear capsule. This lens is held in place by about a hundred tiny threads (zonules), which extend from a muscular tissue between the iris and the retina, called the ciliary body. The ciliary body pulls on these threads or relaxes them to focus the eye. When humans reach the age of forty to forty-five, the lens becomes too stiff to change shape so we lose the ability to focus inward from our natural focus point of clear vision. This lens gradually progresses from being crystal clear at birth, to translucent in mid life, to cloudy, and then opaque with time. This cloudy, or opaque, lens is called a cataract.

The back of the eye is filled with a clear viscous fluid like the thick part of an egg white. This thick fluid is called vitreous. The presence of this material helps to hold the retina in place, but it can be removed without causing a retinal detachment. Once removed, it is replaced with the aqueous humor from the front part of the eye. In later life, usually around age seventy, the vitreous shrinks and eventually pulls loose from the retina. This is called a posterior vitreous detachment (PVD) which is usually harmless. However, the process of separation may rarely cause a retinal detachment.

The back of the eye is lined with two layers. The inner layer is the retina. This is the film in the camera. When light is focused on the retina, the light causes rapid chemical reactions in a layer of cells called rods and cones. The reactions cause electrical pulses in the nerves of the retina. These nerve fibers lead to the optic nerve at the nasal side of the back of the eyeball. They are transported through the optic nerve and tracts to neural pathways to the back of the brain where the occipital cortex makes them into a picture that the brain sees. The chemical process that initiates the neural impulses is very energy dependent and requires a lot of oxygen from the blood.

Behind the retina is a vascular tissue which is filled with dark pigment. This layer furnishes the energy for the retina and clears away the byproducts of the chemical reactions. It is call the choroid. The front edge of the choroid extends past the front edge of the retina as a specialized tissue that contains the ciliary body that focuses the lens and also produces the watery fluid, (aqueous humor) that fills the front of the eye and brings nutrition to the cornea and lens.

Muscles of the Eye
Lateral view

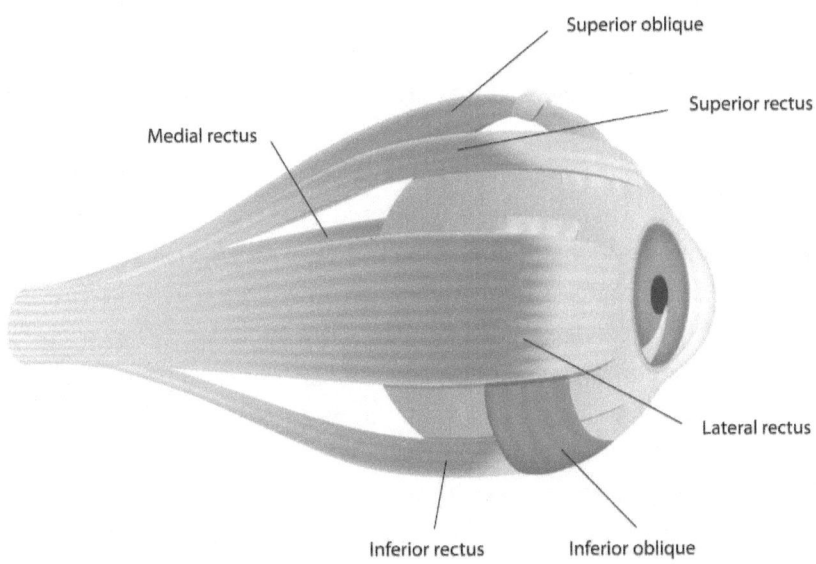

The eyeball is suspended in the eye socket (orbit) by six muscles and many small fibrous bands from the walls of the socket.

Four of these muscles are attached to the bones in the back of the eye socket and insert on the sclera at the top, bottom, right and left sides of the eye. The individual pull of these muscles moves the eye up, down, right, and left respectively. Two additional muscles come from above and below from the nasal side of the eye socket. The superior oblique muscle goes over the top of the eye and attaches to the outside of the eyeball. The inferior oblique muscle passes under the eyeball and attaches to the back and lower outer side of the eyeball. Contraction and relaxation of these muscles rotate the eye around its anterior posterior axis. When the head is tilted slightly to the right or left, the eye rotates to stay upright. Both eyes rotate together so that the pictures from each eye stay aligned.

When these muscles function properly, they receive feedback from the brain to align the pictures that the brain receives from the two eyes so that the pictures merge to form a single, fused image. Malfunction of the muscles or the neurological feedback loop causes double vision, called diplopia. This can be one image above the other, images side by side, or images that are rotationally out of alignment.

The eye socket (orbit), is made up of parts of six different facial bones. The socket is separated from the brain above by thick bone. The rim of the socket is very thick and strong. The nasal and inferior walls of the socket may be paper thin and are susceptible to fracture with trauma. The socket is filled with fat and fibrous connective tissue that hold the eye centered within the socket.

When a fracture occurs in the orbital walls, the fat and fibrous tissues that fill the socket may herniate from the socket into surrounding structures and become trapped, restricting movement of the eye.

The eyebrows rarely cause problems except for aging or trauma. Loss of eyebrows may be the first sign of certain diseases like leprosy and hypothyroidism. The relaxation of the facial skin of the brow, which occurs with aging, may allow the eyelids to sag and put pressure on the upper eyelids to push them down.

Rarely, bushy eyebrows can sag so far that the hairs scratch the cornea. Relaxation of the brow may cause the upper eyelid to fold over and press down on the upper eyelid. The skin may hang over the edge of the eyelid and cover some of the upper field of vision.

Surgical excision of this extra skin is considered medically necessary if sufficient amounts of the upper visual field are blocked by it. Removal of smaller amounts of skin is considered cosmetic and is usually not covered by insurance.

I had a patient who needed surgery for a malignant parotid tumor. The parotid salivary gland is just below the ear and behind the jaw. The facial nerve goes through the middle of it. Removal of his parotid gland tumor caused interruption of the facial nerve giving him a paralysis of that side of his face. His cheek and forehead responded to gravity and drooped. He could not close the side of his mouth and his forehead relaxed so much that his big bushy eyebrows dropped and scratched his cornea. I performed a surgical brow lift, but his continued paralysis allowed the eyebrow to droop again. After that, I had to trim his eyebrows to give him relief.

The skin around the eye is very susceptible to skin cancers, especially basal cell, squamous cell, and adenocarcinoma. Because of the many types of tissue in the eye and eye socket, a wide variety of tumors can originate near, or metastasize to, the eye and the surrounding area.

Eye care providers

I would like to clear up the confusion that most people have about eye care providers. Many people do not know the difference between an ophthalmologist, an optometrist, an optician, an oculist, and an orthoptist. They all begin with "O," but there are definite differences in what care each provider is trained to do and therefore best at providing.

An ophthalmologist is a medical doctor, that is, an MD (medical doctor, allopathic) or DO (doctor of osteopathy, osteopathic).

The training of an ophthalmologist involves sufficient college to gain admission to medical school (usually three or four years), Four years of medical school, an internship for one year, and three years of specialty training in an ophthalmology residency that is approved by the Accreditation Council for Graduate Medical Education. The ophthalmologist is a licensed physician, a medical doctor, who can perform surgery, write prescriptions for all medications, and treat any disease for which he is qualified. Licensure involves a three stage examination by a state board of medicine or the National Board of Medical Examiners. Most hospitals also require ophthalmologists to be certified by the American Board of Ophthalmology in order to obtain and keep hospital privileges.

American Board of Ophthalmology certification requires passing a comprehensive examination covering all of the subspecialty fields of ophthalmology (cataracts, cornea, retina, optics, glaucoma, pathology, etc.).

An optometrist used to be trained to measure patients for, and fit, glasses and contact lenses. Modern schools of optometry teach examination and diagnosis of eye diseases and some surgery of the ocular area, including ophthalmic lasers for myopia in some states. Admission requirements for optometric schools include three or more years of college. Some optometry schools require a baccalaureate degree, but most do not. Graduation from an optometric school as a Doctor of Optometry, an OD (not to be confused with the DO above), requires four years of study and clinical experience in an office or clinic of optometry. After graduation they must become licensed to be able to practice. They can now practice general optometry, or they can go on to do a residency to become a specialist in a field of optometry. The most common specialties are cornea with contact lenses, and pediatric optometry.

The scope of optometric practice is determined by the state legislatures and is usually administered by a State Board of Optometry. Most states limit the medications that optometrists can prescribe and use. They also limit the types of surgery they can perform to minor procedures around the eyes. A few states and the Veterans Administration Hospitals allow optometrists to perform laser surgery for correction of myopia. Some states do not allow optometrists to treat glaucoma, cataracts, macular degeneration or do surgery on the eye as the primary physician.

They can assist ophthalmologists with pre and post operative care. Optometrists have been trying to legislatively expand their scope of practice with regard to the medications they can use and prescribe (including oral and injected medications), and the legal permission to perform surgery, even though they are not physicians.

An optician is licensed to fill prescriptions for glasses, contact lenses, and low vision aids. Some undergo an optional examination for certification by the national Guild of Opticians as an assurance of quality care and they usually advertize that certification if they have it. They can recommend coatings and tints and have liberty to change base curves of the lenses. The measurement of the eye position and position of the pupil is usually left to the optician. These measurements are critical for centering the lens before the eye and the placement of the bifocal, trifocal, or progressive segments in the lenses to allow for near reading and the proper fit of the glasses or contact lenses.

Opticians make and dispense contact lenses. Some contact lenses require special shapes to treat astigmatism and problems with the eyelids. Many opticians are expert at these special lenses. I had the assistance of some very skilled opticians who were able to successfully fit contact lenses for astigmatism and for traumatized eyes that were irregularly shaped after the trauma was repaired.

An oculist in a specialist sometimes called an ocularist, who makes and fits artificial eyes. Some make their own glass, imbed an iris disk, and paint the glass with pigment dusts and glass threads to create an artificial eye that is a perfect mate for the good eye of the patient. My father wore a glass eye from the time he was seventeen years old, but most people did not know that it was artificial.

Modern artificial eyes are made of hard plastic, rather than glass. After an eyeball has been removed and replaced with an implanted sphere, or if an eye has become blind, but is left in place, the oculist shapes the replacement shell that will cover the old eye or the replacement sphere so that it fits snuggly behind the eyelids and moves with the blind eye, or the sphere, so that it follows the other eye and appears natural. If one eye moves and the other is stationery, it immediately looks abnormal.

Another professional that starts with "O" in this field is the orthoptist. These experts work with people with strabismus, which is incorrect alignment of the eyes (i.e. crossed or wall eyes).

They do measurement of the misalignment of the eyes and assist patients with exercises to correct the alignment so that they can use both eyes together and appear normal. Many pediatric ophthalmologists employ orthoptists to teach eye exercises to, and work with, patients who have had recent surgery to straighten their eyes. For some reason, ophthalmologist in England use orthoptists more than ophthalmologists do in the U.S.

Part I

SIGNS AND SYMPTOMS

SIGNS VERSUS SYMPTOMS

There are many things that contribute to the diagnosis of an eye problem. These occur as signs and symptoms. A sign is something which is visible on examination by either the patient or the physician. Symptoms are observations by the patient, a description of what happened and how it feels, or in the case of vision, how it looked to the patient and how it has changed.

One of the most common things I am approached about is pink eye. A friend will say, "Hey, look at this. My eye was kinda red this morning when I looked in the mirror. I was swimming at the "Y" yesterday. Do you think it was the chlorine?"

Red eyes come in several types and severities. I will need to ask if it involves one or both eyes (sign and symptom). Is it getting better or worse? (symptom) Is there a discharge? (sign or symptom)

If so, is it watery, thick, bloody, or have a color? (sign) Does it itch or burn? (symptom) My questions could go on and on.

Symptoms can include: Change of appearance, pain or discomfort, discharge, change in vision including double vision, clouds, shadows, curtains, and haze. They may have sudden onset or be slowly progressive, permanent or transient, affect only near or far vision, be associated with headaches, eating, or menstrual periods. Are there other diseases like hypertension, diabetes, thyroid disease? Some problems are age related.

Change in appearance may mean the appearance of the patient as he looks in the mirror or the change in appearance of objects as they are seen by the patient. One of the scariest things to a patient is suddenly noticing a bright red spot on their conjunctiva.

Usually this is a subconjunctival hemorrhage which may be caused by high blood pressure, coughing, sneezing, vomiting, constipation or heavy lifting. If the blood pressure is normal, we may never know what caused the hemorrhage unless it is correlated with other symptoms like coughing or vomiting.

Vision change comes in many varieties from blurriness, to curtains coming down, to sudden blackout. Some people have a color tint to their vision caused by certain drugs or hemorrhage into the eye. The duration of the visual change is often critical to the treatment. Total blackout from central retinal artery occlusion must be treated within minutes to restore vision, while glaucoma requires years of treatment to maintain vision.

Sudden onset of visual loss seems to happen when something blocks the vision in one eye (the good eye), and the person suddenly notices blurriness, or that a part, or all, of their vision is not there in the other eye. This may cause the sudden discovery of a gradual visual loss.

Some red eyes are painful while others are only mildly uncomfortable or totally painless. Pain is usually associated with serious problems. A red eye from herpes simplex can have a feeling like dust or a lash in the eye, yet it is very serious. As a rule, when an eye is red and has only mild discomfort, the problem is not an emergency. If there is significant pain in a red eye, it may indicate a glaucoma attack, a corneal ulcer, or a laceration of the cornea—all of which are serious problems that require prompt medical attention.

Chronic simple glaucoma is usually painless, has no change in outward appearance, and involves only loss of peripheral vision at first. It may go undetected for a long time until it causes significant damage or is discovered on a routine eye exam. This lack of signs or symptoms has earned glaucoma the name of "the sneak thief of vision." Ophthalmologists recommend a routine check up every two years to check for glaucoma, intraocular tumors, diabetes, and high blood pressure, which are among the many diseases, without symptoms, that can be found in the eye.

RED EYES

I am at a fundraising cocktail party for the History Museum. An acquaintance sees me across the room and decides that it would be a good time to see if I can tell him why his eye has been red for the past three days. He makes his way across the room, stopping briefly to say hello to a few people who recognize him, but he eventually approaches me.

He starts off with small talk, "Hi John, How have you been? Played any golf recently?"

We chit chat for a minute and I notice he has a red eye, his conjunctiva is reddened and his eyes are full of tears, but no pus is caught on his eye lashes. I don't mention any of this since he has not brought it up.

We talk about golf and his recent trip to Denver to visit his aunt. As the conversation starts to lag, he says, "I am glad I saw you here: perhaps you can give me some advice about this eye of mine that has been red for several days."

I give the usual disclaimer that I do not have my usual equipment to take a good look, but I tell him that I can look at his eye and try to diagnose his problem. But first, I need to know more about his red eye.

I ask him, "How long it has been red?"

He says, "Three days."

I then ask if the other eye was red recently. Viral conjunctivitis may affect both eyes at the same time or only one eye. Bacterial conjunctivitis usually involves only one eye. You can get viral pink eye in both eyes, but sometimes the other eye catches it from the first eye during the active part of the disease in the first eye, so the second eye breaks out two weeks later, after the incubation period in the second eye.

He says, "My other eye has been fine."

Pursuing the viral idea, I ask him if he has been around anyone with a red eye, because viral conjunctivitis is very contagious.

He says "No."

It is possible to catch viral conjunctivitis from someone with no signs of the eye infection. Patients are infectious during the two week incubation period after they became infected, but before the eye becomes red and is symptomatic.

I ask him if his eyelids have been stuck together in the morning or during the day.

He answers, "They stick together with dried 'goop' in the morning, but they are watery during the day and I keep wiping them."

Stickiness through the day with a "goopy" discharge would mean bacterial conjunctivitis. Watery discharge, excessive tearing, is typical of allergy and viral disease. He denies any "goopy" discharge during his waking hours.

I take a good look at his eyelids to see if they are swollen or puffy. This can happen with allergic reactions, bacterial or viral conjunctivitis. If the eyelids are swollen and red it is usually bacterial or viral. If they are pale and puffy it is probably an allergic reaction. Allergy usually affects both eyes, but can be from contact of the allergen, like eye drops or makeup, in only one eye.

His eyelids are red and slightly swollen. This puts him in the viral disease category, but it could still be Chlamydia or a very mild bacterial pink eye.

Now things get a little delicate for a cocktail party. I ask him if he has any infections anywhere else on his body. Hey, he asked for the advice! Does he have abscesses, boils, or a draining ear?

Tuberculosis and yeast infections can cause an immune response that causes a small white spot at the edge of the cornea and a conjunctival reaction, creating a red eye.

He replies, "I am as healthy as a horse."

Rather than ask him outright at a cocktail party if he has a venereal disease, I tell him, in a light manner, that I saw a man a few weeks ago who had a red eye from gonorrhea. He says "That's not very likely in my case. I didn't do any messing around in Denver."

At this point I have narrowed down the diagnosis, so I tell him that the most likely cause of his red eye is viral conjunctivitis and that he is very contagious. He may have already given his problem to all of his family, and he may come down with the same thing in his other eye in two weeks. He should not share any towels, handkerchiefs or combs with anyone, should not touch his face with his hands, and try not to touch his wife, or children, with his face or his hands. He should wash his hands frequently throughout the day. Then I tell him that there is no known treatment for this viral disease so it has to run its course.

Now it is decision time for me. Should I tell him that occasionally there is a second phase of this disease that comes on two to three weeks after the red eye clears? This phase involves microscopic infiltrates of the central cornea that feel like there is dust or a hair in the eye and makes the vision slightly hazy, especially in bright light or sunshine. Well, I chicken out and tell him that he needs to be seen by someone with all of the equipment needed to verify my diagnosis. I will let the other ophthalmologist, who is getting paid for his advice, break the bad news to him. He may not get the second phase anyway. He gives me a "thanks a lot" and moves on to talk with someone he has spotted in the crowd.

I head for the restroom to wash my hands so I do not get a red eye or spread his around.

Two common causes of viral conjunctivitis are adenovirus, otherwise known as epidemic keratoconjunctivitis, and Herpes Simplex conjunctivitis. After the first episode of Herpes conjunctivitis, the disease can come back repeatedly as a corneal infection. This is thought to be the result of a partial immunity acquired from the first episode of conjunctivitis.

I saw seven patients in one week who had red eyes, who had come to the emergency room for another reason. All seven had a discharge from their penis which brought them to the hospital. This was diagnosed as Gonorrhea.

The emergency room doctor noticed the red eye on the first patient and called for the eye resident who was on call. When the resident, who had been working with me in the clinic at that time, saw the first patient, he thought the venereal disease was the cause of the red eye also. When he showed me the patient in the exam room the next day, I saw follicles in his lower conjunctiva and noted that he had a red watery eye. I diagnosed this as viral conjunctivitis, and explained to the resident that the patient could have two separate diseases. Gonorrhea in the eye usually causes a very red and swollen eye with a heavy discharge.

All seven men had genital gonorrhea and viral conjunctivitis in their right eye. We were curious why all of them had the redness in the right eye. At the end of the week, a woman came to the clinic with a red eye. She had viral conjunctivitis in her right eye. We wondered if there was another commonality so we asked her about body discharges.

When the answer was positive, we sent her to the gynecology clinic where she was found to have a case of mildly symptomatic genital gonorrhea. We later learned that the first patient managed the motel where the woman was "working." The other men were her clients.

Another cause of pink eye that is sexually transmitted is Chlamydia. In these eyes there is a chronic mildly red eye which can, at times, be purulent. Ocular involvement is usually accompanied by genital or upper respiratory involvement. Systemic medications must be used to control the entire disease process and prevent auto inoculation. Tetracyclines and sulfa medications are the main line of antibiotics for Chlamydia. Tetracyclines must not be given systemically to children because of serious changes to the teeth and bones of the child. I usually gave one medication topically and one systemically. Topical tetracycline in babies and topical sulfa in adults,

Bacterial conjunctivitis is usually very productive of mucoid pus. Some bacteria also cause very red swelling of the eyelids that are often stuck together by dried pus and have to be soaked with warm compresses to separate the eyelids in order to open and look at the eye. Patients with bacterial disease may have a fever, while fever is rare with viral eye disease or allergy.

I have seen advanced cases of allergic reaction to shrimp.

These patients present at the emergency room about an hour after eating shrimp. Many of them knew that they are allergic to shrimp, but they ate them anyway, hoping that they would not react this time. They are often led in to the office or emergency room by a friend, because their eyelids are swollen shut. They are so swollen that it is hard to pry the eyelids apart to examine the eye itself. When the lids are separated, the conjunctiva is usually swollen and glassy looking, but the cornea is usually not affected.

They are treated with BenadrylR and intravenous steroids and usually respond in one to two hours. The emergency room bill usually teaches them not to eat shrimp again, even if they were not scared enough by the reaction.

Allergic reaction is not the only acute reason that people are led into the emergency room. One of the main offenders is often a young man who has been welding or using a cutting torch during the day. He is awakened at one or two o'clock in the night by severe burning pain in both eyes and cannot open his eyes because of the pain. The eye is red and the cornea stains with fluorescein showing the damage from the ultra violet light. These are the signs and symptoms of a welder's burn of the cornea from the ultraviolet light emitted by the arc, or the flame of the torch.

Some of the victims will deny welding without wearing goggles or a welder's hood. I have seen several supervisors who stopped to watch or teach the welder without putting on their own eye protection, saying they did not think they were taking long enough to need protection.

> I had a patient who was a supervisor who was just walking past a man who was up on a ladder cutting some steel on a tank, using a torch. The molten steel hit a flange on the side of the tank and splashed into the supervisor's eye.
> The pain caused a reflex closure of the eye which trapped the liquid steel for several seconds. He sustained a severe burn of the cornea and the inside of his eyelid. The cornea ulcerated and had to be replaced with a corneal transplant. The eyelid had a scar on the inside surface, but it did not bother the transplant.

Other patients who are lead into the office or emergency room with their eyes shut and complaining of severe pain include severe chemical burns and new contact lens wearers who have worn their lenses longer than they should have, or slept in their contacts. One patient who was led into the emergency room had splashed hydrofluoric acid in his eyes and was in severe pain. He recovered to 20/20 vision in both eyes after several weeks.

Some red eyes are caused by diseases that attack the cornea.

The corneal tissue releases substances from the compliment cascade that cause the conjunctival blood vessels to dilate and become red and the eyelids to swell. Machinists and mechanics get small pieces of metal embedded in the cornea. Welders can spray hot metal particles into the eye and cause it to become a red eye. Bacteria infections cause ulcers to develop in the cornea causing a very red, swollen eye which is very painful. The discharge is thick with mucus and pus. People with rheumatoid disease may get a break in the corneal epithelium and quietly melt their cornea away until it perforates, with only slight redness, especially if they have diabetes or vitamin A deficiency. A break or scratch in the corneal epithelium can lead to pain and a red eye, even if there was no infection.

Many patients came to me first thing in the morning, as an emergency, because they woke up at either two o'clock at night or their usual waking time with sudden sharp stabbing pain in one eye. By the time I saw them, they had a mildly red conjunctiva and no visible break in the corneal epithelium. By using back scatter illumination and the magnification of the slit lamp, I could see faint lines and tiny clear cysts; telltale signs of a recent tear which has already started to heal. These are called recurrent erosions.

Often these patients have a history of a scratch to the cornea by something organic—a fingernail, a mascara brush, a stick, or plant leaf. Steel or plastic does not usually cause this problem.

These injuries produce damage to the layer of the cornea that supports the epithelial layer causing the epithelium to stay loosely attached to the cornea rather than heal tightly as it should.

At night, with the eyelids closed, the epithelium swells and, since it does not adhere to the underlying tissue, it forms a blister.

The blister rises through the tear film and may stick to the underside of the eyelid. Movement of the eyelids then tears this blister, exposing bare nerve endings, causing the pain.

The pain upon awakening and opening the eye is understandable, but why at two o'clock, in the middle of the night? We know that dreaming is associated with rapid eye movements—so called rapid eye movement, or REM, sleep. The eyes wobble or shake rapidly, back and forth. When this disrupts the epithelium, the pain awakens the patient. Usually the epithelial tear releases the blister fluid and allows the epithelium to settle down on the cornea and the edges knit back together in a few hours and the pain is gone. This may happen night after night. Therefore, this is called recurrent erosions.

There are many treatments of recurrent erosions including a soft contact lens to hold down the epithelium and separate it from the eyelid, hypertonic salt ointment to draw out the edema and blister fluid as it forms and thereby flatten the epithelium and also to lubricate the eyelid so it does not tear the epithelium.

If this does not work, the ophthalmologist can make tiny prick marks of the involved cornea with the tip of a small hypodermic needle to make holes that the epithelium can grow into to anchor the epithelium. This treatment can be painful and should not be done in the visual area of the cornea. Light scattering scarring may occur at the needle pricks. Another treatment is to have the patient take Librium (chlordiazepoxide), Valium (diazepam) or Dalmane (flurazepam) at bedtime. These drugs will usually stop the REM sleep. These pills are usually used as an adjunct to ointments.

They are all on the addictive list. Usually the epithelium will heal tightly in three to six months, so treatment can be discontinued.

I have had patients who have stopped the treatment too soon and had to start over again.

I have seen several patients with a chronic red eye with no signs of infection. Usually the veins of the conjunctiva are widely dilated and some patients have a dull ache and a throbbing sensation. This is almost always associated with some past significant head trauma—a car accident or a fall with a skull fracture.

Sometimes the patients complain of a whirring sound like machinery. Listening to the skull with a stethoscope sometimes reveals a whirring noise and can locate the problem. When x-ray contrast studies, angiograms of the head, are done, we discover a new direct connection between an artery and a vein that allows high pressure arterial blood to enter the vein, increasing the venous pressure, causing the veins to dilate. This pressure is transmitted to the eye socket and conjunctiva through the ophthalmic vein. Once the neurosurgeons tie off or occlude the connection between the artery and the vein, the vessels return to normal size.

> I have had patients come to me complaining that their eyes are always red. They wake up in the morning with "bloodshot" eyes that stay red all day. They even use eye drops that are supposed to "get the red out." Some of these patients have a watery or slightly mucoid discharge from their eyes. If I look at their eyes with a slit lamp, I may see little nodules in their conjunctiva, but I do not have to look, because they have already told me why they are having this problem.

Eye drops that are formulated to "get the red out" have vasoconstrictors, like tetrahydrozaline hydrochloride and others, to shrink the small vessels of the conjunctiva, changing the redness to pink or white. They work well the first few times they are put into the eye. However, when the effect wears off, the vessels relax and dilate again, often larger than before the drop. The tendency is to put in another drop to remove the redness again.

With repeated use, the drops become less effective and, if they are effective, it is for a shorter period of time. Eventually they do not work and the vessels stay dilated. The conjunctiva reacts to the drops with a follicular response causing the nodules and producing mucus. These whitening drops may help for the photographs of a teary eyed bride or post hangover, but they should not be used for more than a day or two.

RED RIMMED EYES

When the edges of the eyelids become red and tender, it is called blepharitis, the medical term for inflammation of the eyelids. There are many causes of blepharitis and consequently there are many treatments.

Dandruff of the scalp is often associated with scaly flakes in the eyelashes and redness of the lid margins. This is usually not associated with active infection, but is characterized by oily skin of the eyelids and random loss of eyelashes. This is seborrheic blepharitis. It is usually controlled by the use of dandruff shampoo on the scalp, but not the eyelids. Some doctors like to treat the eyelids with baby shampoo, like "No Tears," applied to the eyelids with the finger tips or a cotton tipped applicator, like a Q-tip. In seborrheic blepharitis, the oils of the meibomian glands may break down into free fatty acids that are very irritating to the skin and to the surface of the eye.

Bacteria may colonize the eyelash follicles and the meibomian glands causing a chronic infection and chronic irritation of the eyelids from infectious blepharitis. Pressure on the edge of the eyelid over the tarsal plate may cause a white creamy substance to be extruded from the orifice of the meibomian glands onto the edge of the eyelids. This material is the normal secretion of the meibomian glands that has become contaminated by bacteria in excessive amounts. It comes out of the meibomian glands like tooth paste from the tube.

Much of the irritation to the eye and eyelids is from immune response of the body to the bacteria. Innocuous bacteria can cause this immune response on a chronic basis. When I was a resident, some of the ophthalmologists used allergic desensitization to the bacteria to treat the blepharitis. Another favorite treatment was to give the patient a small pox vaccination. It was thought that the immune response to the vaccination altered the immune response to the bacteria. Getting rid of the normal skin flora (the bacteria that everyone has on their skin and in the hair follicles and sweat glands), is a futile task. The bacteria of the skin are immediately repopulated by contact with people and the world around us.

> I had an older woman as a patient who was receiving chemotherapy for lymphoma. During her course of chemotherapy, she developed blepharitis that itched and burned and occasionally blurred her vision. When I pressed on her eyelids, parallel columns of cerulean blue "toothpaste" came shooting out of her meibomian glands. I knew from the color that it was Pseudomonas bacteria mixed with the oily secretions of the glands. Colonies of these bacteria have this same color on culture plates. The more I pressed on the eyelids, the longer the columns of paste became until they curled around each other.
>
> I treated her with antibiotic ointment, four times each day, applied to the lid margins after first using hot compresses for ten to fifteen minutes. The heat liquefies the secretions and causes them to run out onto the lid margin where the ointment can kill the bacteria. It took three weeks of treatment before I was unable to express the "toothpaste" from her meibomian glands. Tetracycline is one of the few antibiotics that is actively secreted into the glands of the skin. Therefore it is useful in treating bacte rial blepharitis with tetracycline tablets orally, if the bacterium is sensitive to tetracycline.

Children and adults are prone to attract lice to the eyelashes.

The pubic louse is particularly fond of the eyelashes. They appear as tiny particles imbedded within the lashes. On close examination of the lashes, using the magnification of the slit lamp, individual lice can be seen clinging to the lashes. These can be removed by using fine tipped forceps to pull each louse from the lashes or they can be smothered in ophthalmic ointment, either antibiotic or plain petrolatum. The lice lay eggs, or nits, that are firmly attached to the lashes. These are also smothered by the ointment. It is best to continue the ointment for several weeks.

Lice in all body hair must be treated with anti-louse lotions to rid the body of lice. If the scalp, underarms, and pubic areas are not treated, the lice will repopulate the eyelids.

Another cause of red eyelids and a horrendous reaction of the conjunctiva is Stevens Johnson syndrome. This is a systemic allergic reaction to a medication. It involves the entire skin and mucous membranes of the body. The rash appears in coin sized circles or partial circles all over the body. The mucous membranes of the eyes, nose, mouth, throat, gastrointestinal tract and reproductive organs become inflamed, blister, and weep biological fluids. The raw surfaces of the mucous membranes may stick together and scar. The scarring often leads to blindness and, when it was first recognized as an illness, to death in a high percentage of patients who came down with this reaction. With the recognition that it was an immune response, steroid therapy created a very high rate of recovery, but the deformity of mucous membranes and the blindness are devastating. It can be caused by antibiotics, like sulfa and ciprofloxacin, antihistamines like CoricidinR, and a number of other medications.

Treatment of the active stage of Stevens Johnson syndrome requires antibiotic and steroid ointments to the eye and frequent breaking of the adhesions that form between the eyeball and the back side of the eyelids. If these adhesions are not broken, the eyelids will become adherent to the eyeball, covering the eye and keeping it from moving. The eye dries out and the cornea scars and becomes opaque. Once the reaction has healed, the opacity of the cornea may remain, causing blindness. Most of the goblet cells and tear glands of the conjunctiva are usually destroyed, by the disease, leaving a very dry eye.

> An eighty-two-year-old black woman was sent to me after a bout with Steven Johnson syndrome. She had received good care during the illness, but her corneas were both severely scarred and her vision was reduced to counting fingers at about one foot from her eye. While I followed her for the next several months, she developed an ulcer on her right cornea. The ulcer became very deep and her eye started to leak aqueous fluid from her eye through the ulcer. She lived with her daughter, who worked during the day, so she needed better vision.
>
> I tried not to operate on patients with Stevens Johnson syndrome, but the leaking eye forced my hand. I had to do a corneal transplant to her right eye to stop the leak and to save her eye. She also had a dense cataract behind her scarred cornea, so I planned to remove the cataract and replace it with an intraocular lens while I had her cornea open.
>
> She did well after the surgery for several weeks. Her vision improved to about 20/60 so she was able to recognize people and see to get around by herself. She was very pleased. Unfortunately, the epithelium of her transplant broke down because of dryness and she began to ulcerate her transplant. Treatment gradually caused the epithelium to cover the transplant, but the transplant became cloudy and her vision decreased to about 20/400.
>
> She was so happy to be able to see after a year of blindness that she wanted me to do another corneal transplant immediately. The eye was now stable and no

longer leaking and I knew how difficult it is for the cornea to heal after Stevens Johnson syndrome so I convinced her to use the vision she had and not put her eye at risk again.

Another cause of redness of the eyelid margins is contact dermatitis from eye makeup or eye drops. Eye makeup is a major cause of blepharitis. Many of the fancier brands of makeup do not disclose the contents of the makeup. Reading the labels of makeup like Clinique, who does list the ingredients of their makeup, shows that these products are very complicated and contain many different materials—some are organic. Being allergic to any one of these ingredients may cause a reaction.

Mascara that does not contain preservatives, such as chlorbutanol or ethyl and methyl paraben, is a very good culture medium for growing bacteria. Many bacteria grow in small quantities on the eye lashes. When these are wiped onto the mascara brush and placed in the tube of mascara, the bacteria grow and multiply. The next application of mascara will place large numbers of the bacteria back on the lashes. They then invade the lash follicles and meibomian glands of the eyelids to cause infections. Eye shadow and eye liner can also culture bacteria and cause eye infections.

I have seen some nasty scratches on corneas from mascara brushes. Once the epithelium of the cornea is scratched, bacteria can invade the cornea to cause an ulcer. Eye makeup should be replaced frequently to avoid this situation. The manufacturers of makeup are usually reluctant to reveal the contents of their formulas with secret ingredients that make them better than the competition, so it is difficult to tell if they have the antibacterial ingredients. If the ingredients are listed, look for chlorbutanol or the parabens in the list.

While I am on the subject of the rims of the eyelids, I should discuss permanent eye liner. It became popular several years ago to have black lines tattooed along the edges of the upper and lower eyelids. Usually a double row of black dots, very closely together, were drawn just outside the lash line. With these lines, the woman did not need to apply eyeliner pencil along her eyelids.

Unfortunately, the pigment from these black dots occasionally migrated onto the eyelids in some patients, producing a permanent black eye. Tattoos can be removed by laser or skin grafting.

The skin on the eyelid is very thin and skin with that thickness occurs in only a few places on the body. One place is a small area behind the ear and the other is not present in women so that skin area cannot be used for auto grafting of skin to the eyelids. Permanent eye liner has been abandoned by most oculoplastic surgeons.

ITCHY BURNING EYES

I have had patients come into my office, sit down in the chair and, before I have had a chance to ask them what they have come to see me about, they put both fists up to their eyes and grind away at their eyes. I tell them that it is not a good idea to rub their eyes hard like that, but they tell me that their eyes itch so much that they cannot keep from rubbing them.

When I examine them, their eyelids are red along the edges.

Sometimes there are lashes missing. Their conjunctiva has a pale milky look and is slightly swollen. With the slit lamp I can see little bumps in the conjunctiva, behind the lower eyelid, that are called papules. These people are allergic to some airborne irritant.

It is usually pet dander or pollen, but can be dust or some chemical in the air. Their predominant symptom is itching.

Allergic reactions between allergens such as pollens and antibodies, which are made by the body, cause the release of histamine and a host of other inflammatory mediators. Histamine causes blood vessels to dilate and leak serum into the surrounding tissue.

Dilated vessels stretch nerves and cause the itching sensation.

That is why it is best to treat this itching with cold compresses, rather than heat. Cold constricts the vessels and they stop itching.

Heat will dilate the vessels, further aggravating the itching.

The medication therapy consists of antihistamines and vasoconstrictor eye drops. Most vasoconstrictors will not be effective if used more than a few days, so the mainstay of treatment is antihistamines like azalestine (Optivar) or mast cell inhibitors like nedocromil (Alocril). The original mast cell stabilizer, cromalyn sodium (Opticrom), has been on and off the market due to sterility problems in the manufacture.

Patients who present with mainly burning sensation, with only minor itching, usually have a tear film problem causing dry eyes. Either they are not making enough tears to keep the front of their eye moist, or there is some problem with the composition of their tears.

Tears have three main components, water, oil and mucous. The main portion, water, is secreted by the main lacrimal gland in the eye socket and hundreds of tiny tear glands imbedded in the conjunctiva. The mucous portion is secreted by goblet cells in the conjunctiva, and the oil comes from glands on the edges of the eyelids. In a normal functioning eye, the mucous coats the cornea surface and the surface of the conjunctiva of the eye and eyelids.

The mucous allows the water to spread evenly over the surfaces rather than bead up like the water on a freshly waxed car. The oil floats on the outer surface creating surface tension to cause a stable film and retarding evaporation of the water. If there is not enough mucous, water, or oil, the tear film breaks down and creates a dry spot. Small dry spots stimulate the eyelids to blink; large dry spots are uncomfortable to the eye and cause a burning sensation.

Chronic conjunctivitis and certain diseases destroy goblet cells, reducing mucus. Without mucus, the watery tears will not coat the eye, leaving large dry spots.

Blepharitis, which is inflammation of the eyelids, causes excessive oil production. The excess oil adheres to the mucus and causes a film or membrane to form. This also happens if the tear glands do not produce enough water to separate the mucus and oil. The combined oil and mucus produce a film that the eye lids roll into strands that smear on the cornea or float to the nasal cornea of the eye, depending on the amount of tears available to float the strands.

After age forty-five, or menopause, women make fewer tears than men do, on average, and often become symptomatic with foreign body and burning sensations. People, both male and female, with rheumatoid type diseases such as rheumatoid arthritis, lupus, scleroderma, and polyarteritis develop dry eyes. The combination of dry eyes, dry mouth, and a rheumatoid disease is called Sjögren's syndrome. The lacrimal glands and the salivary glands are indistinguishable when viewed under the microscope.

Sjögren's syndrome is so common that there are clubs, nationwide, of people suffering from it. The treatment of dry eyes and dry mouth is difficult. People with Sjögren's have developed tricks and remedies and are eager to share them with other sufferers.

Sjögren's clubs can be found on the internet and in telephone directories. See Teary Eyes, Dry Eyes Chapter.

This is a water deficient type of dry eyes. Because of the lack of water, the tears may have a high concentration of salts and proteins in the tears. This saltiness causes burning in the eyes as the major symptom. These people may benefit from a low salt eye drop, so called hypotonic artificial tears, to dilute the concentrated salt and proteins to stop the burning.

Until recently, the main treatment for dry eyes has been artificial tears, several times a day, to replace the missing tears. This may be augmented by closing the tear ducts which drain the tears from the eye, and the use of soft contact lenses to hold what tears there are against the cornea and conjunctiva to prevent drying.

Several years ago, Cyclosporin A was introduced to treat dry eyes. The popular brand name is RestasisR. Studies showed that the lacrimal glands (tear glands) of dry eye patients were chronically inflamed. This inflammation prevented the tear glands from making tears. Cyclosporin A controls the inflammation and allows the glands to function. Unfortunately, it is expensive and must be used for several weeks before the full effect is obtained.

Cyclosporin A use must be maintained to allow continued tear production.

Burning eyes can be related to other causes. People who smoke cigarettes or are chronically exposed to smoke or other noxious fumes can suffer from burning eyes. People with dry eyes are more subject to irritation than those with copious tears to wash away the offending irritant. This is true of people with chronic blepharitis, inflammation of the eyelids, from both infectious and seborrheic causes.

Chemical injury, both acidic and basic, can cause severe burning sensation in the eyes. This sensation persists long after the offending chemicals have been washed from the eyes. The microscopic damage to the ocular surfaces creates dry spots and the accompanying keratitis (inflammation of the cornea) can persist for weeks. During that healing period, the eyes are very sensitive to noxious fumes, perfumes, smoke and light.

> I had a patient who sustained acid burns to his corneas.
> The surfaces healed to my examination in two weeks, but it was three months before he could tolerate the fumes of his work place. His job was to clean out tank cars before they could be reused. He had not had difficulty doing this before the accident. I got to know him during his treatment and believe that his discomfort was real and not the result of wanting more vacation. On testing he continued to have rapid tear film breakup and the corneal surface stained with dyes that demonstrate damaged tissue. These signs went away at the same time that he reported comfort on the job.

SOMETHING IN MY EYE

One common complaint is the feeling of something in the eye. A piece of dust, an eye lash, or a lint fiber each feel mildly scratchy. Often the discomfort is felt in the area under the upper eyelid, even when the foreign body is on the cornea. Most of these foreign bodies can usually be gently rubbed off with a cotton swab to relieve the discomfort.

I have found some strange foreign bodies in people's eyes.

A four-year-old child was brought in because she was rubbing her eye and it was red. She had been to the beach the day before and had been rubbing her eye since then. When I looked at her with magnification, she had a tiny scallop shell, about one millimeter wide, stuck to the center of her cornea, open side down. It was stuck to the eye like a suction cup and it would not wipe off with a cotton swab.

I managed to tease it off with the tip of a hypodermic needle after I had numbed her eye with topical anesthetic.

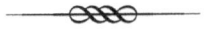

Another small child, about two years old was brought in because his mother could see a small, coppery brown spot in the middle of his cornea. It was very smooth and shiny and did not appear to be on top of the cornea, but rather formed the surface of the cornea. One of the attending surgeons had shown us a lady with a similar brown spot in her cornea. It was an old hemorrhage from abnormal vessels in the cornea. This child did not have any vessels in his cornea to account for the spot. We put the child in a papoose and anesthetized the eye with eye drops. I teased the edge of the spot with a hypodermic needle and the spot popped off. Once I had it in my hand, it looked like the shell of a kernel of popcorn. When the child's mother saw it, she remembered that her children had been eating popcorn at home the day before.

Many problems with the cornea and conjunctiva also feel like something in the eye. A scratch on the cornea, possibly made by a foreign object, will continue to feel like a foreign object until it heals. This feeling may occur intermittently, related to blinking or eye movement, after a foreign body is removed.

Years ago, we would see children and adults with very red eyes.

We would find a speck of dirt or metal embedded in the surface of the eye that was too small to cause a big reaction. Upon further examination, we would find a small tan seed in the conjunctiva behind the lower eyelid. This was a flax seed, put there by their mother or spouse to help remove the foreign body. This was a home remedy. It was suppose to make the eye water so much that it would wash out the offending object. It did not always work and often made the eye much more uncomfortable. I do not recommend putting a flax seed or any other object into the eye for this purpose.

People who do not make sufficient tears often feel like they have a foreign body on the cornea. No foreign body is necessary to cause this sensation. However, having a tear deficiency may cause this sensation by not washing away small, airborne, objects that land on the cornea.

Metal workers and welders may get small pieces of metal embedded in the corneal surface. A windy day will bring patients with small specks of matter stuck to their corneas that must be removed manually. Small particles may become covered with corneal epithelium which causes the sensation to become less or be relieved completely. With lid and eye movement they may later erode through the epithelium and cause irritation until they are covered again. This will recur until the foreign body is removed and the tissue heals.

Patients would come to me saying that they had the feeling of something in their eye. They had been to the emergency room, but the doctor could not find a foreign body. Several days have passed, but they still feel the foreign body, especially when they blink. This is more common that I want to admit. I usually evert the upper eyelid of that eye and find a small fleck of something imbedded in the back of the eyelid. Usually these can be wiped away with a cotton swab and the patient is immediately comfortable.

Most patients who have foreign material on their eye can tell exactly when it got there. When a patient comes to me saying that they have felt like something was in their eye for a day or so, but do not know when it started, I immediately suspect Herpes Simplex infection of the cornea. The herpes virus causes a break in the covering layer, the epithelium. This break has a very characteristic appearance. It takes on the shape of a tree branch so it is called a dendrite from the Greek word for branch. This can be seen with the naked eye by using special lighting techniques, but visualization of the defect is enhanced by eye drops containing fluorescein or Rose Bengal. These dyes glow green in ultraviolet light and pink in white light respectively.

Herpes can occur anywhere in the body and tends to recur in the same place whenever the body is stressed. People respond to many kinds of stress. Fever blisters are herpes of the lips following fever. Excess sunlight, pregnancy, cold weather, other illnesses, and menstrual cycles are some of the common precipitating stresses that induce herpes.

Ocular herpes simplex can involve several parts of the eye, but is most common on the cornea. After the infection, the eye heals, usually without scaring or changes in vision. However, some people have an immune reaction to the virus. This causes a disk shaped area of the central cornea to swell and become hazy. This is called disciform keratitis and it causes damage to the corneal endothelium. It too will run its course and usually clears with return of vision. Each subsequent attack of herpes with the secondary reaction of disciform keratitis results in further damage to the corneal endothelium. Eventually, the corneal edema does not go away because of the accumulated endothelial cell damage. The endothelium becomes leaky, allowing the aqueous humor to leak in to the cornea. The active endothelial process of pumping water from the cornea into the anterior chamber is also decreased, so the edema fluid is not removed from the cornea. The surviving endothelial cells spread to cover the defect so the cornea may slowly recover.

There is an ongoing dispute in ophthalmology about the use of steroids to stop the disciform reaction and prevent this damage.

One school of thought says that steroids reduce the damage to the endothelium so they should be used. The anti steroids school believes that steroids make the viral infection part of the process more invasive. Many doctors defer to both sides so they will treat the viral infection with antiviral drugs and no steroids and then treat the disciform reaction with steroids, covered with antivirals to prevent recurrence of the dendrite.

Sometimes the steroids must be used for several weeks to control the disciform reaction. During this phase, another viral infection may break out on the cornea. Should the steroids be stopped during the active infection? A study by good researchers at Vanderbilt Medical School showed that the eye does better if the steroids are continued while the new infection is treated with antivirals.

If the recurrences are too frequent and destructive of lifestyle, it may be necessary to treat with oral antivirals such as acyclovir or gancyclovir to decrease or prevent recurrence. Patients with

Herpes Simplex of the cornea must be followed closely by an ophthalmologist.

During the spring, both children and adults develop itching and burning eyes with foreign body sensation and watery discharge, usually in both eyes, Because of the time of year this occurs, it is called vernal keratitis and blepharitis. Some patients develop epithelial defects which are refractory to healing and very uncomfortable. Eversion of the eyelids (flipping the eyelid back upon itself, exposing the back side) shows large bumps on the underside of the upper eyelid. These bumps are lymph nodes that become so large that they press against each other and become square bumps with valleys between them. They look like cobblestones.

The first line of treatment is antihistamines, both topical in the eye and systemically with pills. Soft contact lenses may help to heal the epithelial defects and keep them from becoming ulcers. Most children grow out of this problem during puberty.

Some contact lens wearers, both hard and soft lenses, will develop a problem with excessive mucus that smears the lenses and makes them come out spontaneously. The lenses must be cleaned several times each day and the mucus collects on the eye lashes. Eversion of the eye lids of these patients shows the same cobble stone appearance from contiguous papules pressing against each other. This is called GPC for giant papillary conjunctivitis.

It is a reaction to proteins that collect on or within the lens and is more common is soft lens wearers. This is treated with non steroidal inflammatory eye drops with pulses of steroids to quiet flare ups. Changing the contact lenses frequently may avoid recurrences.

> A woman, who was locally famous for her water color paintings, came to me with this problem. She had worn soft contact lenses for years, but had recently been unable to wear them, because of the mucus and the smearing. She was very myopic and did not like to wear her glasses when

she painted. We tried having her discard her soft lenses every week, but the problem returned. About that time, one-day-wear soft lenses were released. She was able to put in a new lens every time she painted and dispose of the lens after one day. This prevented the problem.

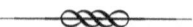

A sweet little Texas lady came into my office one day complaining of having "stickle burrs" in her eyes. Every time she blinked something scratched her eyes. She had tried over the counter lubricating ointments, but the relief was temporary. She had a disease that caused the conjunctiva on the back of her eyelids to shrink, pulling her eye lashes back against her eyes. She also had grown blood vessels into her cornea, which had become scarred and cloudy.

She had a rare disease called ocular cicatricial pemphigoid.

In this disease, the conjunctiva shrinks and the eyelids become attached to the eyeball. The normal structures of the conjunctiva become scarred and misshapen. Eventually the eye cannot move independently of the eyelid.

There is surgical treatment, but the disease is progressive and continues after the surgery. The use of anti metabolites such as Methotrexate and Cyclosporine A may arrest the disease. To stop the lashes rubbing her cornea, they can be epilated to remove them permanently. This involves burning them out by electrolysis, which may be painful. After I removed one lash by electrolysis, my patient decided that she would come to me every three weeks for me to pluck the offending lashes manually. She called it getting a haircut. The lashes could be surgically excised, but she also declined that procedure.

There are other causes of the misdirection of the lashes, called trichiasis. It happens after eyelid scarring from trachoma, eyelid injuries, chemical burns to the eye and chronic infectious blepharitis (infection of the lash follicles). Sometimes a lash just becomes randomly misdirected and scratches with cornea.

Localized red areas on the surface of the eyeball can be benign or malignant. Two common forms of redness that occur in the corners of the eye are the pterygium and the pinguecula. The pterygium is a triangular area of elevated tissue that points toward the cornea and is usually attached at that point to the cornea. It is formed as a healing response to solar damage to the cornea.

Because of its elevation, the eye lid is lifted off of the cornea and does not rub mucus on to the cornea. The water will not coat the bare cornea so a dry spot forms in front of the pterygium, causing further damage. The pterygium tries to heal that damage, growing across the cornea, eventually blocking vision.

If a pterygium starts to grow across the cornea, it should be removed. There are many surgical procedures to use to remove a pterygium; all of them have a high failure rate when it comes to recurrence. Some eyes are treated with Mitomycin C or radiation after a pterygium is removed to prevent recurrence. Some surgeons use conjunctiva tissue, grafted over the excision site or swung as flaps over the exposed sclera where the pterygium was removed.

The other red triangle, the pinguecula, has its base at the edge of the cornea and points into the angle between the eyelids. It is also caused by solar radiation damage to the conjunctiva. These growths may occur in the inner or outer corners of the eye and often occur in both eyes. Treatment with steroids and sun glasses may make it disappear enough to be of no consequence. They can be removed for cosmetic reasons, but healing after removal is disproportionately painful. I have removed them from one eye only to have the patient refuse removal from the other eye because of the pain during healing.

Conjunctiva may become vascularized in local areas with an appearance not typical of pterygia or pinguecula, especially along the limbus, the junction zone between the cornea and the sclera.

This can be carcinoma in situ, a pre invasive malignancy, or it can be invasive squamous cell carcinoma which can invade the eye and spread throughout the orbit (eye socket).

Other diseases such as gout, uveitis (inflammation within the eyeball), and blepharitis (inflammation of the eyelids) can cause red eyes. They will be discussed in other chapters.

TEARY EYES, DRY EYES

I learned of a patient, when I was a resident, who came to their eye doctor complaining that she could no longer cry. The ophthalmologist took her quite literally and did a workup for tear function. He found that she did not make many tears and had a relatively dry eye. She did not make more tears when the eye was irritated. He told her to take artificial tears three or four times a day and come back to see him in one month. She immediately went home and committed suicide. The doctor had missed this woman's plea for help with her depression. Apparently, her symptom of being unable to cry was to tell the doctor that she wanted to cry because she was depressed, but could not cry, because of her dry eyes. The added diagnosis of dry eyes may have increased her depression. This inability of her physician to see her depression may have been what pushed her over the edge.

I saw many patients with dry eyes. Most were very frustrated by their dry eyes, but none were clinically depressed. Many patients who are starting to have decreased tear production will complain of excessive tearing from time to time. This is because, when the eye becomes slightly dry, the conjunctiva senses this dryness before it becomes irritating. This subconscious signal causes the nervous system to switch on the main tear glands, flooding the eye with tears. These tears overflow the eyelids and blur the vision which is noticeable to the person.

Studies have shown that premenopausal women make more tears than men of the same age. However, after menopause, the hormonal changes cause a decrease in tear production, causing many women to complain of dry eyes. Tear production decreases with age in both sexes, so many men develop dry eyes in their seventies and eighties. Patients who have worn contact lenses for many years will notice the dryness because of discomfort with their contact lenses. Hard lenses need a tear pool to float over the cornea. With decrease tear volume and increased salt concentration, soft contact lenses lose some of their water content, causing the edges to curl. This is irritating to the eyelids as they blink over the lenses. Many contact wearers can tolerate this by using artificial tears as often as needed to augment the tear film and rehydrate their soft lenses. People who have worn contact lenses for many years have been shown to have decreased corneal sensitivity and awareness of the dryness that stimulates more tears.

One major cause of dry eyes is rheumatoid arthritis or another rheumatoid type disease. Apparently, the inflammatory disease attacks the salivary and the tear glands in addition to the joint and other collagen structures in the body. Rheumatoid diseases include scleroderma, systemic lupus erythematosus, ankylosing spondylitis, polyarteritis nodosa, and dermatomyositis. Some doctors include Chron's Disease. All of these diseases can lead to Sjögren's syndrome, which is dry mouth and dry eyes, combined with a rheumatoid disease. This is a very refractory type of dry eyes. Dryness of mucous membranes is not confined to the mouth.

Many people with Sjögren's syndrome have difficulty swallowing, painfully dry nasal passages, constipation, and vaginal dryness.

People with Sjögren's syndrome have developed ways to ease these problems. Sugarless lemon drops and glycerin swabs ease the oral dryness. Vaginal suppositories containing Nystatin can be used in the mouth to treat the thrush infection of the throat that happens in the dry mucous membranes. Sugary sweets must be avoided to prevent rapid tooth decay that is enhanced by the lack of saliva. There is a national organization, the Sjögren's Syndrome Foundation, with chapters across the country that helps people cope with these problems. They publish a newsletter with important information about Sjögren's syndrome survival.

The Foundation can be contacted at www.sjogrens.org. or at Sjögren's Syndrome Foundation, 6707 Democracy Blvd. Suite 325, Bethesda, MD 20817.

Many cases of dry eyes are caused, or exacerbated, by medications being taken for other diseases. Neuropsychiatric drugs like Librium and Valium decrease tear production. Many antihypertensive medicines, bladder control drugs and even multi-day underarm antiperspirants can cause dry eye symptoms. Your ophthalmologist can help sort out any medications that may contribute to dry eye symptoms. Often another drug can be substituted for the offending one. If not, the symptoms may be ameliorated by the usual treatments for dry eyes.

Treatment of dry eyes is based on replacement of the lost tears.

Artificial tears are sufficient therapy for the majority of dry eyed patients. Closure of the drainage tubes that carry tears from the eyes into the nasal passages, using either punctum plugs, thermal cautery, or laser burns, helps to keep tears in the eyes. RestasisR, a brand of Cyclosporine A, is a popular, but expensive, treatment.

It suppresses inflammation in the lacrimal (tear) glands, allowing them to make tears again.

As the drying becomes chronic, the surface of the eye may break down and become rough and hazy. Strands of epithelium tear loose forming filaments which feel like small, sharp rocks in the eye. People with this problem may benefit from soft bandage lenses and frequent artificial tears. The soft lens holds the artificial tears in the eye and over the cornea. The affinity of bacteria for the soft lens in a dry eye makes the eye more susceptible to the complication of infection. Sometimes antibiotic eye drops must accompany the artificial tears and soft lens to avoid infection.

Severe dry eyes may be treated by sewing the eyelids together, except for a small gap in the center which allows vision straight ahead. This is called a tarsorrhaphy. The small opening leaves a minimal area for evaporation. Sewing the nasal ends of the lids together decreases the flow of tears to the tear ducts that drain the eye.

Wearing swim goggles creates a moist chamber in front of the eyes, decreasing tear evaporation. However, the trapped moisture may fog the goggles and obscure vision. Wiping the inside of the goggles with a silicone cloth will cause the moisture to bead and run off of the lenses, leaving the vision clearer. These silicone cloths are available at sports stores where they are sold for use on ski goggles

While I was at Massachusetts Eye and Ear Infirmary, Dr. Marshal Doane invented a device that would slowly pump artificial tears through a tube into the eye. The device could deliver about three milliliters of tears in twenty-four hours, which is slightly more than the normal amount of tears produced in a day.

The pump was a glass syringe with an electrolytic chamber in the plunger. Electricity from a battery created a slow electrolytic gas formation. This build up of gas forced the plunger down the barrel of the syringe at an imperceptible rate creating a very minimal flow of artificial tears. The glass reservoir in the pump had to be refilled every three days using sterile techniques. The tubing from the pump could be run behind the ear and along a spectacle frame and into the space behind the eyelid. It was a cumbersome system with many drawbacks, but the patients who used it thought it was wonderful.

Another device that was invented to supply tears to the eye used an ink jet printer head that was mounted on spectacle frames to spray tears onto the cornea many times each minute. This mist often fogged the spectacles used to hold it, so it was not practical if glasses were required. The frames without lenses worked well, if vision was good enough, or the discomfort was very bad and the patient placed comfort over vision, so foggy lenses did not matter.

Fortunately, only a few of the most severe cases require this level of treatment.

LUMPS AND BUMPS AROUND THE EYE

Swelling around the eye is easily seen, especially if it is localized.

Bumps in, or under, the skin of the eyelids can be benign or malignant. Two common benign bumps on the eyelids are the cyst, also called a chalazion, and the sty, also called a hordeolum.

The chalazion is a blocked oil gland of the eyelid, called the meibomian gland. There are about twenty-five meibomian glands in each lower eyelid and fifty glands in each upper eyelid. When they become blocked by infection or plugged secretions, the oils that they secrete are trapped in the gland and cause it to swell and create an abscess. This stretched tissue is painful. Treated with warm compresses, five minutes, three or four times a day, the abscess within the chalazion will liquefy and point to the surface, open, and drain itself, usually to the posterior surface of the eye lid. An egg may be hard boiled and wrapped in a wash cloth to hold over the chalazion. This egg holds heat better than a wet washcloth. It can be reheated and reused, but should not be eaten after the treatment is finished. The bump will go away in a few days to two weeks.

If the treatment does not cause the cyst to drain, the bump may persist for up to a year. People who are inpatient can have them drained surgically. The incision to drain the abscess is made on the inside of the eyelid and does not leave a scar. The gland is removed through the incision using a curette to scrape out the glandular tissue. Once this is removed, it will usually not recur.

However, new chalazia may form in the remaining glands.

The hordeolum is a plugged meibomian gland that is infected or blocked at the point where the gland empties onto the edge of the eyelash follicle. The eyelid may point out from the edge at this location. These can be expressed by squeezing with cotton swabs, or opened with a small needle to permit drainage, but neither of these treatments is recommended. Hordeola are best treated with hot compresses, like a chalazion, to promote spontaneous drainage. If they do not resolve with compresses, they can be opened surgically to drain the abscess.

Antibiotics are rarely indicated for either the chalazion or the hordeolum since they are usually not infected and antibiotics are ineffective against abscesses. Abscesses must be drained, surgically or spontaneously, or they will slowly reabsorb. If the eyelid becomes red and swollen, the abscess may be infected, in which case antibiotics must be added to the treatment in addition to the compresses. Drainage will allow rapid clearing of the infection.

The eyelids are frequent locations for both squamous cell carcinoma and basal cell carcinoma. A rare eyelid tumor, adenocarcinoma of the eyelid, involves the meibomian glands of the eye lids.

Adenocarcinoma of the eyelid is often misdiagnosed because the can be mistaken for a chalazion, however, they may be aggressive and metastasize early to distant organs where they become lethal.

The squamous cell carcinoma spreads locally and can metastasize to distant parts of the body. The basal cell carcinoma does not usually metastasize, but can spread locally by extension. It can invade the orbit, the surrounding bone, and the brain.

All three of these tumors should be removed by an ophthalmic plastic surgeon. The most urgent is the adenocarcinoma, followed by the squamous cell carcinoma that may metastasize. The basal cell tumor can be watched for growth, or signs of invasion, before removal is necessary. Smaller tumors are easier to remove and leave small scars and require less reconstruction. Because the facial skin is so prone to cancer, sunscreen or makeup with sunscreen should always be worn in the summer sunlight. Cancer of the eyelids may require Mohs surgery, a procedure to remove the tumor layer by layer and examine the edges to be sure that no tumor is left behind to allow recurrence.

Melanoma, a pigmented skin cancer, may arise from the skin of the eyelids. It appears as a freckle, but continues to grow and become thicker to the touch. Freckles are normal around the eyes and on the iris within the eye. If a freckle changes color, becoming darker, or begins to spread from its original size, it should be examined by a dermatologist to determine whether it should be removed. Melanoma has a tendency to metastasize to other organs within the body, especially the liver, and can lead to death.

Mohs surgery is recommended for the removal of melanomas.

Senile keratoses of the eyelid look like basal cell carcinomas, but grow much faster. Both tumors have a crater in the center which may fill with keratin from the skin over the tumor. Although they are benign, they should usually be removed if they interfere with normal eyelid function. They are considered precancerous, so they must be watched closely if they are not removed.

Molluscum contagiosum usually occur in children. A molluscum is a raised bump with a crater in the center which is filled with a cheesy substance. Removal of the cheesy substance with a curette makes the lump go away.

The skin of the eyelids and face is susceptible to common warts and neurofibroma, as in Von Recklinghausen's disease—neurofibromatosis.

Systemic lupus erythematosus usually called Lupus, can cause the formation of a nodule on the eye lid surface. The presence of the systemic disease leads to the diagnosis of a lupus nodule. They come and go, but they can be removed for cosmetic reasons.

Leprosy can manifest as a lump on the eyelid. It can cause loss of eye lashes and eye brows, saddle nose, and uveitis.

> While doing eye care on the Island of Montserrat, a lady came to the clinic with a very large mass on her upper eyelid. This mass was so large that she could not open her eye. I helped Dr. Sterrer remove that mass in one piece by dissecting the skin from over it and shelling it out from a depression in the tarsal plate. She had a saddle nose and many skin areas that had lost all pigment, a typical sign of leprosy. When we asked the local nurses how common leprosy was on the island, the said that there had never been a case on the island and refused to order testing for it on this lady. Unfortunately, there was not a pathologist on the island to examine the mass we removed to settle the question whether or not it was leprosy.

SWELLING

The skin around the eyelids is loosely attached to the underlying bone and muscles so it is susceptible to swelling and is slow to resolve that swelling. Allergic reactions lead to rapid swelling which is very soft and puffy. Hypothyroid disease causes infiltration of the tissues to form a doughy swelling around the eyes. Finger pressure on a small area of this swelling will leave a dent that can persist for several minutes. Hyperthyroid disease causes infiltration of the eye socket and the muscles around the eye, which cause the eye to protrude forward in an eye bulging stare.

People with kidney disease, who retain fluid, develop swelling throughout the body. Because of the ease with which the eyelids swell, it may be noticed first around the eyes.

Tumors within the eye socket displace the fat which surrounds the eyeball and push against the eyeball or the eyelids. Dermoid tumors are benign and can occur in various positions within the eye socket. They cause local bulges in the eyelids and can displace the eyeball and turn it away from its intended direction of gaze.

Tumors of the optic nerve, such as meningiomas and optic nerve gliomas push the eye forward. These may occur independently or in association with Neurofibromatosis (Von Recklinghausen's disease). Rhabdomyosaroma, a tumor that affects children, can occur anywhere in the orbit and presents as displacement of the eyeball away from the tumor and forward. Metastases of cancers from other parts of the body can occur in the eye socket and become apparent when they grow and displace the eyeball.

When my wife was a pediatric intern, she called me to see a four-year-old black child who was brought in because his eyes protruded. The pediatricians were worried about hyperthyroid disease or renal failure. The child was normally active for a four-year-old and was not over or under weight for his age. His eyes protruded forward with the center of the eyeball slightly forward of the outer edge of the eye socket, one of the criteria for exophthalmos, the eye protrusion from thyroid disease. The pediatricians had ordered all of the tests for thyroid disease and renal function so I agreed to follow the little boy with them. I stopped by the floor that evening to check with my wife about when she would be ready to leave. I saw that the child's parents who were there to visit their son. Both the mother and the father had very protruding eyes. I went to the library to look up the differential diagnosis of ocular proptosis (protrusion) and discovered that a rare cause was familial shallow orbit (eye socket) syndrome which is hereditary. When all of the lab tests came back normal, I realized that this child had the rare occurrence of familial shallow orbit syndrome, which is considered a normal variant, not a disease.

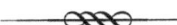

This reminds me of a night on call during my residency when the emergency room doctor called me to ask if I was familiar with "Froggy the Gremlin." I was half awake, but I said I had heard of him in some story. The ER doctor told me that "Froggy" was in the emergency room and wanted me to come take a look.

In the ER, I saw a black woman, who was about twenty five years old. Her eyes were both sticking out past her eyelids so that she could not close her eyes. Her eyelids were trapped behind her eyeballs. I asked her how this happened and if this was the first time it had happened.

She said that she had done it before, but that this was the first time she could not press on her eyes and make them go back in the sockets. She had bilateral ocular prolapse.

She said that she was riding on a bus when another lady was yelling at her for something she had done, so she decided to "freak out" the other lady by popping out her eyes. It had the desired effect, causing the other lady to leave the bus. When she tried to close her eyes again, she could not get her eyes back into the sockets, so she came to the emergency room.

I tried pulling on her eyelids, but they were trapped behind her eyes. I finally anesthetized here eyes with eye drops, put on gloves, and pushed her eyes back into their sockets with my thumbs. I checked her vision and it was unaffected by her prank. I advised her not to do it again because she could stretch her optic nerves and loose her vision. She said that she would not do it again because of the discomfort and the difficulty getting them back to normal.

CROSSED EYES, WALL EYES, AND DOUBLE VISION

The mechanisms that control the movement of the eyes and make them work together are very complex. They involve the six muscles that move each eye, the vision or picture from each eye, the middle ear, many connections within the brain, as well as the conditions around each eyeball. These factors can be involved in many types of trauma and different diseases such as high blood pressure, stroke, thyroid disease, and diabetes.

Some children are born with, or acquire during infancy, the inability to align both eyes on the same object. I will deal with these problems with ocular alignment in children in a separate chapter. Children with strabismus, the failure to align the eyes, may go into adulthood with the same or residual problems from their early disease. Here I will address acquired alignment problems in the older child and the adult.

Sudden onset of double vision in the adult is usually a result of problems of the nerves and muscles that move the eye, or the brainstem, the part of the brain that controls them. There are four muscles, the rectus muscles, which mainly move the eye up, down, right, and left. There are two more oblique muscles that rotate the eye around the line of vision and come into play when looking to the corners of vision. These six muscles are controlled by three nerves to each eye.

One nerve, the oculomotor nerve, or third cranial nerve, goes to four of the muscles, the three rectus muscles that move the eye up, down, or toward the nose, and the lower rotator muscle, the inferior oblique. This nerve also controls the muscle that opens the upper eyelid, the levator muscle, and it also controls the size of the pupil.

The fourth cranial nerve, also known as the trochlear nerve, goes to the upper rotator muscle, the superior oblique.

The sixth cranial nerve, called the abducens nerve, goes to the abductor muscle, the lateral rectus muscle that moves the eye away from the nose.

All of these muscles are controlled by brain segments (nuclei) within the brainstem, the base of the brain. Those nuclei receive signals from various parts of the brain including cerebral cortex (vision center), the cerebellum (balance center), the middle ear (equilibrium center), and the proprioceptors (muscle sensing nerves) of the legs. Input from all of these areas facilitates the alignment of the eyes.

Third Nerve Palsy: A relatively common occurrence in people with either high blood pressure or diabetes is a paralysis of the third cranial nerve. This is caused by damage to the nerve from a vascular accident. The nerve has a blood supply that can be interrupted by closure of the capillaries into the nerve. Both hypertension (high blood pressure) and diabetes can cause these capillaries to close, damaging the nerve. When the third nerve is damaged, the muscles controlled by it become flaccid and relax.

The eye will be pulled away from the affected muscles so it turns out and down because the lateral muscle and the superior oblique still have muscle tone, but the others are paralyzed. The muscle that lifts the eyelid is also paralyzed so the eyelid is closed. The pupil may dilate in the affected eye, but usually does not. This usually happens to only one eye at a time.

> I had an old gentlemen come into the clinic complaining that he could not open his left eye since he woke up that

morning. When I opened his eye to look at, his eye was turned down and outward. He then complained that he saw double and wanted to know what I had done to him to cause that. He had not tried to open his eye before this and had not realized that the muscles that move his eye were paralyzed. He was sure that I had caused his double vision. He had both diabetes and hypertension to cause his paralysis.

Another cause of third nerve palsy is an intracranial aneurysm.

A common location for an aneurysm is at the major branching of the internal carotid artery as it forms part of the Circle of Willis. Smaller arteries connect the carotid artery to the posterior cerebral artery and also connect the two anterior branches of the internal carotid artery (the anterior cerebral arteries) to form a ring of arteries around the base of the brain called the Circle of Willis. This gives redundancy to the blood supply to the brain by connecting all of the arteries that make up the circle.

These branches are very near the spot where the third cranial nerve emerges from the brain stem and runs along the arteries.

Pressure on the nerve from a bulging sacular aneurysm from any of these arteries can cause paralysis of the third nerve. The nerve fibers that control the pupil are in a band that lies on the outside of the nerve and are very susceptible to pressure from an aneurysm.

Therefore third nerve paralysis from an aneurysm is usually accompanied by a dilated pupil.

Third nerve paralysis from diabetes or hypertension involves the feeder vessels of the nerve and usually does not affect the pupil. This is an important distinction. Patients who are suspected of having an aneurysm should be seen immediately by a neurologist or neurosurgeon. They may need immediate surgery to clamp the aneurysm. Patients who have normal pupil responses should be seen by an internist, within a week, to be checked and possibly treated for their diabetes or hypertension.

Hemorrhage inside the skull can cause the brain to shift and produce pressure on the nerves giving the same effects. There are many unusual causes of third nerve palsy including brain tumors, multiple sclerosis, thyroid disease, stroke, migraine, and viral diseases such as chicken pox, measles, shingles, and several other rarer diseases.

Myasthenia gravis may present like a third nerve palsy, but the cause is muscular, rather than neuronal. The distinguishing characteristic of myasthenia is the inconsistency of the paralysis. It may involve one muscle on one day and another muscle the next day. The paralysis tends to fatigue and become more pronounced with extended testing.

Fourth nerve palsy: The sudden occurrence of vertical double vision (one image above the other but also displaced horizontally (right or left) and sometimes rotated so that the two images appear rotated with respect to each other is because of paralysis of the fourth cranial nerve. The forth nerve, also called the trochlear nerve, enervates the trochlear (superior oblique) muscle. This muscle is attached to the posterior eye wall of the eye socket and travels forward to the upper inner corner of the eye socket where it passes through a ring, like a pulley, and turns toward the eye. It attaches to the top and the back of the eye. The pull of this muscle causes the eye to rotate down and out, away from the nose.

Paralysis of this nerve removes this force and allows the inferior oblique muscle to pull the eye up and out without the opposition of the paralyzed superior oblique muscle. Since the oblique muscles also rotate the eye to keep it level and aligned with the opposite eye, the inferior oblique will rotate the eye with the top moving away from the nose.

The major causes of for a fourth nerve palsy include vascular diseases like diabetes, high blood pressure, and trauma. Tumors, aneurysms and hemorrhages can block the nerve. Local or generalized inflammatory processes such as meningitis, sinusitis, polyneuritis, as well as viral systemic diseases like measles, and herpes zoster interfere with the nerve function.

Bilateral fourth nerve palsy can be secondary to trauma when the person is thrown forward in an automobile accident, helmet to helmet head-on collision, or over the handle bars of a bicycle striking the forehead straight on. This causes the brain to surge forward in the head pushing the fourth nerves against the Tentorium Cerebelli, the membrane that holds the brain in place within the skull. This can bruise or sever the nerves.

Sixth nerve palsy: A patient who develops the turning of one or both eyes toward the nose and is unable to turn the eye outward has a paralysis of the sixth cranial (abducens) nerve(s).

The abducens nerve and muscle pull the eye outward. When it is recently paralyzed, the eye will follow an object from the nasal side toward the outside until it reaches straight ahead, but will go no further. If the opposing muscle, the medial rectus, is not paralyzed, it will have some contraction tone and pull against the paralyzed muscle, pulling the eye toward the nose. If the nerve has been paralyzed for days, or weeks, the medial rectus muscle will contract preventing the eye to go to the midline (straight ahead). The double vision here is horizontal (side by side) unless other nerves are involved.

Trauma and vascular problems, such as stroke and diabetes are common causes of double vision. Each cranial nerve arises from a nucleus within the brain. These nuclei depend on blood vessels for their oxygen and nutrients. A stroke or local disease which blocks these vessels will cause the nuclei to lose control of the eye muscles leading to double vision. Whenever the eyes do not work together, the cerebral mechanism for depth perception will not work and the world loses its depth or three dimensional appearance. Blockage of the vessels to the brain centers for the intracranial nerves are often associated with loss of other functions that cause other signs of stroke such as paralysis of arms and legs, inability to speak clearly, think straight or see large segments of the normal vision area. Combinations of symptoms may indicate where the vessel is blocked and which portions of the brain are affected by the stroke. Tumors pressing on brain nuclei can be located by what functions are affected.

People with major stokes may not be able to see anything to the right or the left in either eye, depending on the side of the stroke. They lose vision toward their paralyzed side. This complicates physical therapy, because it allows them to ignore the paralyzed limbs.

Another frequent cause of sixth cranial nerve palsies is elevated intracranial pressure from bleeding, tumors, and pseudotumor cerebrii.

Pseudotumor cerebrii is a disease in which the brain makes too much cerebral spinal fluid, the fluid that surrounds and protects the brain. This fluid is made inside the brain to fill the meningeal space around the brain and flows through and around the brain and spinal cord. It exits at the base of the spinal cord and is reabsorbed there. In pseudo tumor, the spinal fluid is made faster that it is eliminated so pressure builds within the skull, causing a headache.

Increased intracranial pressure prompts a thorough examination for a brain tumor. Pseudotumor is a diagnosis of exclusion.

In pseudotumor, all tests and neurological examinations are negative for a brain tumor except for bilateral sixth nerve palsies, if they are present. The sixth nerve has a long course from the brain stem to where it exits the skull and may be susceptible to pressure compressing its blood supply. The pressure causes headaches, dizziness, blurred vision, double vision (from crossed eyes), and transient visual obscurations (blackouts).

This disease is most common in young obese women with irregular menstrual periods and can be aggravated by caffeine, pregnancy and birth control pills, tetracycline, and Vitamin A excess, among other rare suspected causes.

All of the reasons just stated for double vision are based on the two eyes not looking at the same place. There are other causes that produce double vision in one eye (monocular diplopia.)

These include uncorrected near sightedness (myopia), cataract, high astigmatism, and corneal irregularities such as scarring or keratoconus.

> A thirty-five-year-old woman came to see me because she was seeing double tail lights on the cars ahead of her and she thought she had a brain tumor, or something like it, making her see double. She also thought that she needed new glasses because her glasses were five years old and everything far away was getting blurred. When I examined her, I found that she had become more nearsighted since her glasses were fitted. I checked the alignment of her eyes and did not find anything abnormal. Knowing that under corrected nearsightedness could cause double vision, I asked her to check for double vision with her new glasses and call me if she still had it. She did not call me so I assume that the double vision went away. Maybe she thought I was a quack and did not bother to call.

Corneal scars can scatter light creating a second image that looks like a shadow of the first image. Glasses and contact lenses will not make the shadow disappear. A new cornea (cornea transplant) will correct the problem, but most people will learn to ignore the shadow image and avoid the risks of complications that may follow a corneal transplant.

Both men and women may develop a thinning of the central cornea at about the age of puberty. The pressure in the eye causes this thinned cornea to bulge outward making the cornea slightly conical rather than the correct spherical shape. This is called keratoconus. This cone shape is often pointed downward or to one side. This irregular conical cornea does not focus the light on the retina so the vision is blurred or double vision occurs.

When the bulge is slight, a hard contact lens can be fit to vault over the bulging cornea to give a new spherical shape to the front surface of the eye. That new surface now bends the light, correcting the irregularity and focusing the light correctly on the retina.

If the cone protrudes too much, the contact cannot ride correctly and falls out frequently. Once the cone reaches this stage, the usual treatment is some form of corneal transplant. The type of transplant has changed and become somewhat controversial over the past ten years and there is also work being done on collagen cross linking to shrink the cone back to a better shape without a transplant.

DROOPY EYELIDS, PTOSIS

A fifty-five-year-old housewife came in to see me because she was having trouble keeping her eyes open. She said that it occurred in the afternoon and evening. She said that sometimes it bothered her left eye and sometimes her right eye. She did not know how to predict which eye would bother her and it did not happen every day. She also complained of double vision which came and went at odd times. When I examined her, I had her look up at my light which I held high in front of her. At first, her eyelids lifted with her pupil so she could see my light. As I held the light high, her eyelids slowly drooped until they covered her pupil and she could not see the light. This is typical of myasthenia gravis, a disease caused by failure of the nerves to communicate with muscles.

Myasthenia often causes eye muscle problems before it is diagnosed in other parts of the body. It can be confined to the eye muscles. If it spreads to the body, it may become life threatening, requiring frequent medications to maintain breathing and other body functions.

Drooping of the eyelid is called Ptosis. It can be caused by problems with the nerves to the upper eyelid, muscle injury or malfunction, or malformation of the eyelid. Children may be born with ptosis or develop it shortly after birth. These will be covered in the children's part of the book.

A young man came into the clinic complaining of drooping of his left eyelid. This had slowly progressed over several months. He denied trauma to his eye or his head. Our plastic surgery expert saw him and decided that his levator muscle, the muscle that opens the eye, had been stretched and that he needed surgery to correct his ptosis. The surgery consisted of everting the eyelid, exposing the levator muscle, and cutting some of the muscle out to shorten it so it would lift the eyelid.

When the surgeons exposed the muscle, a contact lens popped out of the opening. It had cut through the levator muscle and become embedded in the eyelid. The surgeon reattached the severed muscle where the lens had cut through it. When we asked the young man about this after the surgery, he told us that he had lost a contact lens about a year before. He had knocked it off center and then could not find it. He thought it had fallen from his eye and he had lost it. After the surgery he did well.

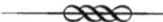

A fifty-six-year-old man came to see me one day because he had noticed that his left eyelid was always lower than his right one. I looked at him and noticed that this was true; his left eyelid was about two millimeters lower than his right. This was true on up and down gaze. The left eyelid was resting just above his pupil while his right eyelid was just covering the edge of his cornea and visible iris, near the sclera. I also noted that the pupil on the left side was smaller than his right pupil.

When these two signs show up together, there is usually absence of sweating on the same side of the face. Together these are called Horner's syndrome, which occurs when there is injury to the sympathetic nervous system component of the third cranial nerve. This pathway leaves the brain and travels down the spinal cord to the neck where it exits and forms a string of nerve nodes along the carotid artery as it returns to the head. Neck injuries to the spinal cord, carotid artery or spine are frequent causes of this. Cancer of the top of the lung, spreading into the neck, can also cause this picture.

BLOWOUT FRACTURE

A fourteen-year-old boy was brought to my office after being hit in the right eye by a racket ball. His eye was swollen shut, but after several minutes of pressure with a cold compress, he was able to open the eye enough that I could check his eye and his ability to move the eye. The eye looked normal, but his vision was blurred. He had mild edema (swelling) of the retina which explained his poor vision. He could move the eye to the right and left and look down. When he tried to look up the eye stopped just above straight ahead and could not look up. He reported that he saw double whenever he looked up. When I placed anesthetic drops in his eye to numb it and grasped his eye with a forceps, I could not move the eye upward. It was as if he had a wire holding his eye from going up. When I pulled the eye to the "end of the wire," it stopped moving.

He had what is known as a blow out fracture of the orbit or eye socket. I sent him for X-rays of the bones around the eye.

This fracture involves some of the paper-thin bones that form the walls of the orbit or eye socket. The thinnest bones are the wall between the orbit and the nasal passages and the bone between the orbit and the maxillary sinus which is the hollow space between the orbit and the roof of the mouth. When an object, which is larger than the front opening of the orbit (a ball or fist, for instance), strikes the eye and covers the orbit entrance, it compressed the contents of the orbit and increases the pressure on these thin bones, causing them to crack. The fat in the orbit may be pushed into these cracks and become wedged in these cracks as they close when the pressure is released after the blow.

Within the orbital fat, there are ligaments which attach to the muscles that move the eye. These ligaments or the muscle itself may become trapped in the cracks, restraining the movement of that muscle and the eye. Surgery is necessary to remove the muscle and ligaments from the cracks and repair the fracture so that the ligaments and muscles do not become trapped again.

This requires surgery which could endanger the eye, so it is controversial. Many ophthalmologists will not operate if the patient does not have double vision when looking straight ahead.

Because of damage to the muscle, the patient may wind up with double vision after surgery, even when double vision was not present before the surgery. Excess pressure on the eyeball during surgery of the eye socket may compromise the blood supply to the retina and cause blindness. If there has been extensive damage to the fat around the eye, the eye may sink in the socket, making it difficult for the brain to point it the same direction as the fellow eye. This causes a double vision which is very hard to correct.

When I repaired blowout fractures, I placed a plate of silicone on the floor of the socket to close the hole and slightly elevate the eyeball. I did not see double vision in these cases. The volume of the implant probably compensated for fat loss from the trauma.

Blowout fractures involving the nasal wall of the eye socket are more difficult to repair because of the attachment of the ends the eyelids to the rim of the socket on the nasal side. They can be repaired if the entrapment is causing side by side double vision, but are otherwise left alone to heal.

Automobile and industrial accidents, bar brawls, and sports trauma to the face may cause fractures of the bones around the eye socket. The bones make a continuous structure around the eyeball so fractures though the rim in one place are often accompanied by a fracture elsewhere to allow the bone to move away from the trauma. Since the zygomatic arch, the bone at the side of the face, which runs from in front of the ear and attaches to the rim of the eye socket, is attached to the orbital rim, it is often fractured at the same time. Large sections of the orbital walls may be detached from the skull forming a free section of bone. When this includes the floor of the socket, the bone fragment may settle below the usual position, allowing the eye to sink in the socket.

This makes the eye look up to see the same thing that is straight ahead on the other eye. This unusual view, although only slightly different from the view of the other eye, makes it difficult for the brain to align the two eyes. Usually the bone fragment must be realigned surgically and stabilized to the surrounding bones to repair this problem.

A severe blow to the eye from a ball, fist, dash board or other object may cause damage to the eye. This may affect the retina, the pupil or the lens in the eye. After an eye injury, the compression and release of pressure in the eye may cause retina to swell distorting the alignment of the rods and cones and making the retina pale and hazy. Strong forces can break the capillaries in the retina and cause hemorrhages which block the light to the retina beneath the hemorrhage. This condition has the fancy name, *commotio retinae*.

If the retina tears, it can hemorrhage and fill the eye with blood. This blood may form a blood clot within the vitreous gel, or be diffusely spread throughout the vitreous. Small amounts will cause red, or pink, colored vision. A large clot may block vision completely or have dim red vision when a strong light is shown into the eye. Diffuse hemorrhage will slowly clear over several days to weeks. Clots may dissolve and clear over weeks.

Clots may go on to organize into an intraocular membrane within the vitreous, blocking vision. This membrane may contract as it matures over weeks or months and eventually pull the retina loose from the choroid tissue beneath it leading to a full-blown retinal detachment. This membrane must be removed before it causes the detachment. A surgical procedure, developed in the late 1960's and early 1970's, called vitrectomy uses an instrument with a small needle containing a cutting blade and suction tube to nibble the membrane without pulling on it and thereby causing a retinal detachment.

A blow to the eye may cause the retina to tear along the attachment at the front of the eye with only minimal hemorrhage. This retina edge will gradually peel loose from the choroid and may progress to a total retinal detachment. The progression of the detachment appears to the patient as a shadow or curtain which slowly moves across the vision in that eye over hours to days. This is a very serious problem which must be treated immediately to avoid permanent loss of vision. Treatment of retinal detachments will be discussed in a separate chapter.

PAIN

There are many kinds of pain in and around the eye. There is a dull aching pain which may not be apparent when the person is distracted. There is sharp stabbing pain, sometimes associated with blinking, that will awaken a person from deep sleep. Some eye pain is associated with bright light. A dull pain around the eye may be exacerbated by eye movement, looking to the right or left.

> A fifty-year-old woman came to me with the complaint of a dull aching pain that she felt in front of her eyes. She said that the pain was not in her eye, but that it came from about an inch in front of it. There are no nerves hovering in space in front of the eye, but that is where she located the pain. This pain often happened after she had been reading in a darkened room with a table lamp for light.

This pain can occur with acute glaucoma or uncontrolled chronic glaucoma. I examined her looking for signs of acute glaucoma.

This is a condition in which the iris moves forward in the eye to cover the outflow channels from the eye. These channels are located at the edge of the cornea where it meets the sclera.

The iris is attached to the ciliary body on the inside of the sclera where the sclera meets the cornea. The flat iris forms an angle with the dome of the cornea, called the angle, which is usually about 45 degrees.

Farsighted people have shorter eyes, so the lens and iris are sometimes pushed forward, narrowing this angle from the usual 45 degrees to only 10 to 15 degrees. When the pupil dilates, the iris bunches up near its attachment to the sclera, blocking the outflow channels. This happens in dim light, like when watching television in a dark room. The treatment is to use eye drops to constrict the pupil, pulling the iris away from the outflow channels, thereby pulling the angle open.

This attack can also happen in very bright light or after prolonged reading when the pupil becomes very small. The small pupil pulls the iris tight against the lens of the eye and blocks the flow of aqueous humor from the ciliary body, behind the iris where the aqueous fluid is made, through the pupil to the anterior chamber in front of the iris where it escapes from the eye.

This blockage creates pressure on the back side of the iris, pushing it forward against the outflow channels, blocking them. The treatment here is to moderately dilate the pupil to relieve the blocked flow of aqueous humor which will allow the iris to fall back, and opening the angle.

Once the pressure increases, it blocks the blood flow to the muscles in the iris, weakening them. When this happens, the drops are not effective in moving the pupil, either dilating or constricting.

If the acute glaucoma attack cannot be stopped with medications, a hole, called a peripheral iridectomy, must be made through the iris near its attachment to the ciliary body and sclera.

When I started practice, this was done by cutting through the edge of the cornea, pushing on the eye to expel some iris through the opening, cutting a hole in this exposed iris, and then milking the iris back into the eye, being sure that the red reflection from the retina showed through the hole in the iris to prove that the hole was open all the way through the iris. The incision was usually closed with one stitch.

With the invention of ocular surgery lasers, it became possible to burn a hole through the iris without making an incision in the cornea. The laser light is focused in a cone shape so that it comes to a point with high energy. This light is shown through the cornea while being directed at a thin part of the iris. Then the point of the light is focused on the iris using a low energy focusing laser beam, the high powered laser is fired and a hole is burned through the iris. If the hole is all of the way through, a cloud of pigment bursts through the hole. The pigment comes from the back side of the iris, proving that the hole is open. The success of the burn is reinforced if the red light reflection from the retina can be seen through the hole.

A variation of this mechanism of angle closure, called malignant glaucoma, occurs after cataract surgery. Once the lens has been removed, the vitreous may come forward and block the pupil. This does not occur very often now because the intraocular lens that has been placed in the capsule bag pushes the lens and bag posteriorly, holding it away from the pupil. However pressure from the vitreous can push the lens and bag forward and block the flow of aqueous through the pupil. This will increase the pressure in the eye very rapidly, causing severe pain. Dilation of the pupil with eye drops should break the blockage and lower the pressure. If this does not relieve the pressure, the vitreous face must be cut with a needle knife to release the vitreous pressure and allow the lens and capsule to fall away from the pupil to release the blockage. The knife is introduced through the cataract incision line and is directed through the iris toward the center of the eye to release fluid trapped in the vitreous.

> But I digress. The lady, who came to see me, did not have the elevated pressure of glaucoma when I saw her. She did not have a narrow angle. This is normal, but it also the case between glaucoma attacks. People with narrow angles may have many small attacks that resolve spontaneously before having a major attack. I told this lady that I wanted her to come in to see me while she was having the pain before her eyes.

About three weeks later I got a call from her, saying that she had a headache in front of her eyes. I told her to come in immediately. When she arrived, her eye looked normal, her iris was back and her pupil was slightly dilated.

Her pressure was elevated to 35 mmHg (millimeters of mercury). (Normal is 10 to 21.) When I put the special gonioscopy lens on her eye to look back into the angle, I found it was closed for the full 360 degrees. The central iris was well back from the cornea, but a peripheral ring of iris had fallen forward, covering the outflow channels. This was happening in both eyes. She had what we call a plateau iris. It was flat, but the peripheral iris had closed the angle.

I put pilocarpine eye drops into both eyes, and in 30 minutes her pupils were small and her pressure had dropped to 15 mmHg. I put the gonioscopy lens back in each eye and determined that the angle was now open, 360 degrees in both eyes. I told her to use 1% (weak) pilocarpine drops in each eye twice each day to keep the angle open, but return immediately if she got the same type of headache again. I also advised her to have holes (iridotomies) made in her iris in both eyes so that she could quit the pilocarpine eye drops. She took my advice and was cured.

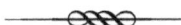

A young man was led into the emergency room by his girl friend at midnight one night when I was on call. He said that he had severe pain in both eyes that was so bad that he could not open his eyes when there was light, even in a dimly lighted room. This is such a frequent occurrence that I asked him if he had been doing any welding.

He told me that he was learning to arc weld at work and had welded all day. My next question was whether he had worked in his helmet and eye shield all the time. He told me that he forgot to put it on after lunch for about ten minutes until his supervisor saw him and told him to put it on. He had a welder's burn from severe ultra violet light that had burned both corneas like severe sunburn. He was treated with patching of both eyes and given a sleeping pill to take when he got home to sleep it off. His girl friend led him home.

If he had been a woman of the same age, I would have asked her if she had new contact lenses or had over worn her old lenses.

Over wearing of hard contact lenses causes the same symptoms, but it is caused by oxygen deprivation of the corneal surface (epithelium), The cornea has more nerve endings per square millimeter than any other part or the body. When it is injured by scratching, foreign bodies, oxygen deprivation, or chemical injury it is extremely painful with burning or stabbing pain.

Another cause of acute onset of pain is corneal hydrops from keratoconus. In keratoconus, the central cornea becomes thin and may stretch because of the pressure within the eye. This stretching may then cause Descemet's membrane, on the back surface of the cornea, to split. Since the endothelium adheres to Descemet's membrane it is also split. This creates an opening in the barrier that keeps aqueous humor, the fluid in the eye, from entering the cornea. Once the split has occurred, the fluid rapidly enters the cornea and the cornea swells. Epithelial edema follows, creating blisters in the corneal epithelium which break, tearing the epithelium and exposing nerve endings. The damage to the epithelium and the swelling of the cornea are both very painful.

The endothelium will eventually heal and form a new barrier to the fluid, stopping the corneal edema and relieving the pain. The usual treatment is to patch the eye with a firm eye pad to relieve the pain until the endothelium can heal. In severe cases with very large tears, a penetrating keratoplasty may be necessary to repair the cornea.

In my experience, corneal hydrops occurs more often in keratoconus related to trisomy 21, called Down's syndrome. This is probably because of the reluctance to operate on Down's syndrome patients who have a higher risk of rejection and injury to the cornea. I have done many transplants on high functioning Down's syndrome patients, but usually prefer not to operate lower functioning patients because of their inability to understand and cooperate with the protection of the transplant.

Inflammation inside the eye, caused by infection or noninfectious uveitis, causes a dull aching, unrelenting pain in the eye. Much of the pain comes from irritation of the iris and ciliary body.

Infection in the eye, called endophthalmitis, causes significant dull boring pain. It usually follows a penetrating injury, or surgery, to the eye. It can happen rarely by spread through the blood stream from an infection elsewhere in the body like an abscess or prostatitis. Intraocular infection with bacteria and viruses occurs commonly in AIDS patients. This type of infection, through the blood stream, is called metastatic endophthalmitis.

> A young musician came to the emergency room in Galveston one night with a high fever and chills. The emergency room physician diagnosed him as having sepsis, infection in the blood stream. Blood cultures were taken and he was started on intravenous antibiotics. He got nervous and ducked out of the emergency room and disappeared. Two weeks later he came to the clinic complaining of a painful red left eye with blurred vision in that eye. The resident who examined him dilated his pupil and looked into the eye. He saw several small fuzzy white balls that looked like cotton floating in the vitreous

gel in the eye, near the surface of the retina. These were typical of infection within the eye that has come from the blood vessels.

When the resident learned that the musician had been in the emergency room he called for the laboratory results and learned that the blood cultures had grown a fungus, Candida Albicans. To treat this he required two weeks of intravenous infusion with the antifungal, Amphotericin B, which meant hospitalization for two weeks.

He was a young, healthy man with no obvious source of fungus infection serious enough to enter his blood stream. He was in Galveston playing in a rock band at a local hotel. He and the rest of the band were living in a room at the hotel with their pet dog. He denied intravenous drug use. When one of the band members visited him in the hospital, he told us that the band all used intravenous drugs. He went on to explain that he had stolen some of our patient's drugs and did not want him to know about it so he drew up some of the water from the dogs bowl into a syringe and injected it into the drug bottle to restore the lost volume. We had no way of knowing what was in the dogs bowl two weeks before, but there was a good bet that it had some Candida Albicans.

The musician's eye improved rapidly and the cotton balls disappeared. The treatment regimen called for two weeks of medication, but on about the tenth day he disappeared from the hospital, leaving his intravenous behind.

We checked with the hotel and learned that the band had left town the day he disappeared. He probably went with them to the next gig. We never heard from him again. No doctor inquired about his treatment in Galveston. He was probably cured by ten days of treatment.

With modern techniques of cataract surgery, most patients feel little or no pain and what little there is usually abates within hours. If a patient comes in complaining of pain in the next few days, it is usually an indication of high pressure in the eye, or an abnormally soft eye because of leakage from the incision. Severe pain is most commonly from an infection within the eye. If the pressure in the eye is not high or low, the pain is usually caused by infection inside of the eye. Some infections are low grade, caused by bacteria that usually do not cause much trouble. The more pathogenic bacteria like Staphylococcus or Pseudomonas can proceed to destruction of the eye within hours to days. They must be treated aggressively with intraocular injections of antibiotics and steroids.

> A woman called my office on a Monday morning, wanting to be seen immediately because her eye was very painful.
>
> She explained to my receptionist that she had her cataract removed on Friday and she was in severe pain. She had called her ophthalmologist on Sunday about the pain and he told her to take two Tylenol, and that he did not need to see her on Sunday. The pain had gotten worse after the Tylenol, so she had lost faith in her surgeon and wanted to see me.
>
> I saw her that morning. She could barely open her eye because of the pain and light sensitivity. When I put in anesthetic drops and opened her eye, it was very red.
>
> Her iris was very grey except for large corkscrew vessels bulging from it. In fifteen years of seeing infected eyes, I had never seen corkscrew vessels before. The aqueous fluid in her eye had congealed and it had many white blood cells imbedded in it. Usually when there are blood cells in the aqueous, they float around like dust in the sunshine.
>
> When they do not move, it means that the aqueous has congealed from the high concentration of protein

that has leaked from the dilated blood vessels. This solid aqueous was beginning to form a white membrane on the front of the intraocular lens that had been inserted behind the pupil during surgery. Because of this membrane, I could not see behind the lens into the back of the eye.

I made up high concentration antibiotic eye drops and ordered strong steroid eye drops for her to put into the eye every hour and asked her to call me by 5:00 PM to tell me how she was doing. Usually when we are using the right antibiotic, there is relief of pain within eight hours. She called just before 5:00 PM to tell me that she was much more comfortable. I had her continue her eye drops and come to see me again the next day.

When I saw her the next day, she told me that the pain was completely gone. This made me think that this was a reaction to something during surgery and not an infection.

I decreased her eye drops to every four hours for the next week. By that time, the aqueous gel became liquid again and the white blood cells disappeared. The blood vessels shrank back, straightened, and withdrew into the iris tissue.

The membrane on the surface of the intraocular lens became dense white and I discovered another membrane on the back surface of the lens. These two membranes blocked her vision from that eye. I decided to wait several weeks for the eye to settle down from the reaction before opening the membranes with the YAG laser to restore her vision.

Six weeks after the surgery, I took her to the laser room and cut holes in the membranes with the laser. I checked her vision and it was very good. That evening she called me at home to tell me that the pain was returning to her eye. I told her to come to the office early in the morning.

The next morning she had a red eye with gelled aqueous, white blood cells and a faint membrane on her lens.

The iris vessels were dilated, but not as bad as before. I started the same regimen of eye drops as before and she again obtained relief within hours.

Several months before, I had heard a presentation about a bacterium, Micrococcus, which caused mild infections within the eye. That particular bacterium produces faint bull's-eye rings on the implant lens. The rings are made of a protective coating that covers the bacteria and keeps the white blood cells and the antibiotics from killing the bacteria. The bacteria become dormant within this coating and do not cause a problem unless the coating is disturbed.

The only sign of a problem was low grade inflammation in the eye which can last for weeks or months.

I decided that the original cause of her pain was infection with Micrococcus that had become dormant, surrounded by the protective coating and incorporated in the membranes. When I disrupted the membrane and the protective coating, it released the bacteria and started the inflammation all over again. To avoid another repeat, I had to kill the bacteria before I reopened the new membranes.

This bacterium is sensitive to the antibiotics chloramphenicol and clindamycin when given as pills.

Chloramphenicol had a bad reputation for causing aplastic anemia, which is often fatal, so it was no longer being used. Clindamycin had killed a number of older, debilitated patients by giving them mucous colitis and diarrhea, several years before. Since that epidemic of deaths from clindamycin, it had been discovered that the mechanism of death had been the antibiotic killing of the normal bacteria in the gastrointestinal tract. The patients affected by this were found to have clostridia bacteria, which were not sensitive to clindamycin, growing in their gall bladders.

Without the inhibition of the normal bacteria, the clostridia grew rapidly and caused the diarrhea that killed the old debilitated patients.

My patient was in her sixties, working, and in good health. I explained the problem with clindamycin and told her there was a chance of a diarrhea problem. She said that she was willing to take the antibiotic to get rid of her eye problem and would stop if it gave her loose bowels.

That afternoon, I received a frantic phone call from the patient's sister. She told me she was a nurse and wanted to know why I was trying to kill her sister with clindamycin.

She said that I should call her sister immediately to tell her to stop the mediation. When I called the patient, she told me to ignore her sister, she wanted to take the medicine and cure her eye.

She took the medicine for a week and came back to see me. She had experienced "a touch" of diarrhea, but kept on taking the clindamycin. She felt fine. A week later, I repeated the laser treatment, restoring her vision, and she did not have any reaction.

I moved to Pittsburgh several months after caring for her. She wrote me a letter a few months later saying that she wanted to come to Pittsburgh for me to remove her cataract. I wrote to her, giving her the names of two good ophthalmologists, other than her first surgeon, and told her she would be happier at home after the surgery. She wrote to me several months later to tell me that her second cataract surgery had gone smoothly.

Small imperfections or foreign particles on the cornea may be slightly irritating or cause severe stabbing pain. They are usually more painful when rubbed by the eyelid during normal blinking.

A twenty-seven-year-old woman came into my office complaining that she had pain and a scratchy sensation in her left eye for several days. She had been to the emergency room two days before and was examined by the doctor using a slit lamp. He told her that she did not have anything in her eye and that she had probably scratched it and it was healing, but she might still feel like something was in her eye. After two more days, she was still feeling something scratch her eye.

I looked at her with the slit lamp and put fluorescein dye in her eye to look for scratches on the cornea, which would stain with the dye. She had several small vertical scratches on the cornea which should have been healed if there were not a foreign body present. This was a dead giveaway that there was something under her eyelid that scratched her cornea every time she blinked. I twisted a paper clip open to a figure eight and used it to evert her eyelid so I could see the back side. (the long edge of one end of the paperclip was laid on the upper eyelid, above and parallel to the lid crease. With the other hand a bunch of eye lashes are grasped between thumb and forefinger.

With the patient looking down, the lashes are pulled up and outward until the eyelid flips onto the paper clip. This exposes the back of the eyelid.) I could see a small black spot imbedded in the underside of her eyelid. I grabbed a cotton tipped applicator and wiped it away. When I let the eyelid flip closed, she blinked a few times and told me that the scratchy feeling was gone.

For some reason, many doctors are reluctant to evert the eyelid to look for the foreign body behind the eyelid when it is not obvious on the front of the eye. Everting the eyelid is mildly uncomfortable for the patient, but it is necessary to find the foreign body.

The eye is not very good at localizing pain. A person with a foreign body, embedded in the cornea or conjunctiva will usually localize that pain source as on the upper cornea or under the upper eyelid, even when the object is embedded in the lower cornea or the nasal or temporal conjunctiva. When a foreign body is removed from the cornea, leaving a divot in the cell layer that covers the cornea, some discomfort often remains until the divot is covered with new epithelium. This usually takes from one to twenty-four hours.

When an iron foreign body is embedded in the cornea for more than several hours, the iron molecules diffuse around the foreign body and are absorbed into the cornea. Over the next twenty-four hours, these particles oxidize to form rust. This rust forms a plaque around the site of the foreign body and will remain there for many months unless it is physically removed.

This is accomplished by teasing a small needle under the plaque and lifting it loose, or by grinding away the plaque with a rotating burr. The divot left in the anterior corneal stroma fills in with epithelial tissue restoring the smooth surface of the cornea.

Copper and brass may do the same thing. Stainless steel does not form plaques.

> I had another woman who as in her fifties who complained of a dull aching pain in both eyes that bothered her constantly and was getting worse. It was so bad that she could not sleep at night and she was suffering from sleep deprivation. She said it was worse when she looked to either side. At first it was relieved by mild pressure on her eyes, but now it hurt her to touch her eyes. When I examined her, I could not find any physical changes to

account for her pain. This is typical of posterior scleritis, which is inflammation of the white outer coat of the eye.

Scleritis is thought to be related to rheumatoid diseases and is treated with systemic nonsteroidal anti-inflammatory drug such as aspirin, and ibuprofen. Some cases require treatment with anti metabolites, such as anticancer drugs, to stop the pain.

This same type of pain can occur with choroiditis, inflammation of the pigmented, vascular layer of tissue between the retina and the sclera. This is usually caused by viruses, bacteria, fungi, and parasites, such as measles, tuberculosis, syphilis, histoplasmosis, and toxoplasmosis to name a few. Non infectious causes include autoimmune diseases like Behcet's disease, periarteritis nodosa, and malignancies like leukemia and reticulum cell sarcoma.

Sarcoidosis can also cause choroiditis. Choroiditis of many forms is more common in patients with AIDS.

Another form of choroiditis presents with very mild discomfort in the eyes after reading and the inability to focus on near objects in patients who are less than forty years old and not presbyopic (cannot focus because of the age of their lens). The cause is anterior uveitis, also known as pars planitis, named after the part of the anterior choroid from which it arises. This is mostly a disease of unknown cause that occurs in young people. This disease is often asymptomatic and will run its course over five to ten years. In symptomatic cases it can be helped with topical steroids.

However chronic use of steroids runs the risk of glaucoma and cataracts, caused by the steroids.

Photophobia is a special form of pain that is brought on by light entering the eye. It is caused by injury or infection of the cornea, inflammation within the eye, and meningeal irritation such as meningitis, bleeding from the brain, migraine headache, or trauma to the meninges. The meninges are the protective membranes that surround the brain.

Injury to the cornea includes medication induced keratitis (inflammation of the cornea), conjunctivitis, corneal scratches or ulcers, and corneal edema. These require specific therapy for the particular problem.

Inflammation in the eye can be from iritis (inflammation of the iris), uveitis (inflammation of the choroid, ciliary body and iris), or infection of the retina and vitreous. All of these are serious and need the attention of an ophthalmologist to sort out and treat correctly.

Causes of meningeal irritation may be determined by examination and related symptoms or a history of head trauma, either open or closed. I have seen chronic photophobia from a skull fracture which entrapped the meninges in the fracture. For entrapment of meninges in fracture lines, an MRI may be necessary to make the diagnosis.

> A sixty-year-old widow came to see me complaining of severe pain that caused her to keep her eyes closed most of the time. She said it burned and felt rough when she blinked her eye. She told me that she could not go out anywhere with her friends because of the pain. She was missing church and could not play bridge. She had rheumatoid arthritis, but it did not interfere with her getting around.
>
> All the time she was sitting in the exam chair, she had a hand over her eyes and held her head down. I had to put anesthetic drops into her eyes so that she could open them so I could examine her. The anesthetic drops did relieve her pain. This told me that it was a surface problem. One look at her told me that she had very dry eyes. Another ophthalmologist had started her on artificial tears to relieve the dryness. She said the drops were almost worthless.
>
> They only relieve her pain for a few minutes.

The surface of her eyes was dull and looked like etched glass. There was no layer of tears along the lower eyelid for the lids to spread over the cornea. Her conjunctiva looked like leather and was reddened. She was very dry.

I put bandage contact lenses in both eyes to hold any tears over the cornea and increased her artificial tear drops to every two hours or more often if she felt dry between drops. When she came back in a week the bandage lenses were still in her eyes, but she still kept her eyes closed and her head down. The redness was gone from her conjunctiva.

The cornea had lost its etched glass appearance.

She said that she was still miserable. She still had to stay at home in the dark. The physical signs were much improved, but she would not admit to feeling any better.

This went on for several weeks with continued improvement of the appearance of her eyes, but no improvement in her symptoms.

One day I took my family to a local cafeteria for dinner and spotted her ahead of me in line. She had her eyes open and was chatting with a friend as she went through the line. She did not see me. I noticed that she sat with her friend and carried on a conversation with her throughout dinner and walked out without ever covering her eyes from the overhead fluorescent lights.

When she next came to see me, about two weeks after I saw her at the cafeteria, she was covering her eyes and complaining that what I had done for her had not helped her. I advised her that she should continue the lenses and tear drops and that she would slowly improve. I did not embarrass her by telling her that I had seen her at the restaurant when she did not appear to have any problem.

About a month after that, I went to the Catholic hospital across the street from the medical center to see a consult.

When I walked into the lobby of the hospital, I was surprised to see my patient sitting behind the information desk, looking up patient room numbers for visitors. I could not resist walking up to her and saying hello. There were two other ladies at the desk so she did not cover her eyes and act like she was in pain, since she had been acting very normal before I arrived. I complimented her on her progress and the fact that she was volunteering in the community. She never pretended to be in pain after that. I am sure that her pain, when she first saw me, was genuine, but that it had gone away with the therapy. Books describe a rheumatoid personality that is very negative toward admitting improvement.

One disease that does not cause pain or other symptoms until the late stages is glaucoma. It often goes undetected because the damage is being done with no pain or other symptom.

In what is called chronic simple glaucoma, the pressure raises so gradually that it does not cause pain. The damage done to the optic nerve usually affects the peripheral vision, to which we do not pay much attention in daily life. If a person starts bumping into cupboard doors or low branches, it may draw attention to the loss of peripheral vision. This loss shows up as cuts or scars on the forehead. The last vision to go in advanced glaucoma is the small central area and a small temporal area. Since one eye is usually affected before the other, the loss of visual field is often masked by the good visual field and normal vision in the good eye.

Almost all vision may be lost in one eye before the person notices.

I saw a lady on the island of Montserrat who was brought in by her daughter, because she could not see well enough to drive. She had to search for almost two minutes to find the eye chart on the wall, but she read the 20/30 line when she finally found it. She had never had pain in her eyes, but she could no longer see to drive. When I tested her, she could only see an area less than five degrees wide in either eye. Her pressures were in the mid thirties and she had no pain. Her optic nerves were cupped out to bean pot shape, because of the elevated pressure had blown them out, destroying the optic nerves.

Because glaucoma does not have any pain or other symptom to draw attention to it, the only way to discover it in the early stages is to have a routine eye exam by an ophthalmologist.

During the exam the pressure in the eye is measured and the optic nerve is examined to see if there is typical damage to the nerve by the high pressure. The pressure causes the center part of the nerve to die, leaving a pit or cup in the center of the nerve where it exits the eye via a hole in the sclera. The pressure on the nerve, against the edge of the hole in the sclera, blocks the capillary flow of blood to the nerve and the flow of cellular fluid within the nerve. The combination permanently kills the nerve fibers. See the chapter on Glaucoma.

Ophthalmologists are often sent patients who complain of headaches. In my experience, very few headaches are caused by poor vision. The vast majority are caused by stress. Reading under stress may cause a headache, even with proper glasses.

Occasionally we find a person who had significant uncorrected astigmatism. The distortion is so great that they have to struggle to read, especially if the reading involves fine print or poor lighting on the page. Correction of the astigmatism with glasses or contact lenses may relieve this type of headache which manifests as tired eyes and aching around the eyes.

People in their forties, who find themselves holding what they are reading at arm's length and having trouble reading, even at that distance, may have presbyopia, which is the inability to focus in close due to age. These people will benefit from reading glasses or bifocals if they already use glasses for distance vision. I recommend simple reading glasses from the drug store for those people who do not need glasses for distance vision. To select the correct power, take a piece of the want ad section of the newspaper with you and try the different powers on the rack until you find one that you can read the want ads at a distance of about ten inches from your nose. Then you can read comfortably at the recommended distance of fourteen inches for a long period of time.

Most people start at +1.25 or +1.5 and progress every year or so through +2.0 and then +2.5. This power, +2.50, is good enough for most people for the rest of their lives.

> One type of headache may affect vision very dramatically.
>
> I had a frantic call on a Monday morning from one of the nuns at St. Francis wanting to be seen right away. She had been seen on Sunday in the emergency room for symptoms of rainbow colored flashing lights in the center of her vision. After she had the flashing lights for awhile, she developed a severe headache. She was seen by a neurologist.
>
> They had done a CAT scan of her brain which was read as normal.
>
> I asked her to describe the flashing lights. She told me that they were multicolored and looked like rainbows in their color distribution. She told me that they moved around and swirled around her central vision. Then everything got very dark in the center of her vision and she could not see except for her peripheral vision.
>
> I went to the library in the clinic and pulled a book from the shelf. It was Walsh's book on neuro-ophthalmology.
>
> I opened it to a page of colored photographs and showed it to her. She gasped, "That's it. That is just what I

saw." I told her that she had a classic ophthalmic migraine headache. It is caused by vascular spasm in the cerebral cortex, the part of the brain that interprets the signals from the eye into vision.

I have had ophthalmic migraine headaches with the same flashing, swirling, colored lights. I was in an antique store in New Orleans looking at antique chandeliers with rows of prisms. Then I noticed that I was seeing prismatic rainbows on everything. I stepped outside of the shop and saw prismatic rainbows on everything I looked at. Then I noticed a small dark spot in the center of the prismatic light. I knew that some people lose vision entirely for a brief period of time and cannot drive a car or read while they have the symptoms, so I paid close attention to the blind spot. It did not grow, but it began to disappear in about ten minutes. Twenty minutes later the visual disturbances were all gone and I started to get a headache.

Ocular migraine headaches are very disturbing to people, especially their first one. I have had several patients draw pictures of what they saw. They usually match the drawings printed in Dr. Walsh's Textbook of Neuro Ophthalmology. Usually we do not treat them unless they become numerous and interfere with the person's lifestyle. They can be treated like regular migraine headaches.

I usually send the patient to a neurologist who is familiar with treating migraine headaches for their treatment.

FLASHES AND FLOATERS, CURTAINS AND SHADOWS

The appearance of flashing lights and/or black spots drifting around in front of you is one of the true emergencies in ophthalmology. I have had emergency room doctors make up stories about the patient having flashes and floaters, just to get me to see someone right away.

Flashes in the peripheral vision, sometimes described as fireworks going off, are the response of the retina to being touched, pulled, or torn. The vitreous jelly that fills the back of the eye liquefies with age. The long chain molecules of the glycose aminoglycans that compose the vitreous are tightly folded like a wad of string. With time, and especially in the presence of diabetes, the molecules unravel and are broken up by enzymes. The remnants of this enzymatic digestion are reabsorbed and disappear. People over sixty years old lose part of their vitreous by reabsorbtion. The fibers that course through the vitreous begin to shrink once the filler is gone. This places traction of the back of the vitreous body.

The posterior surface of the vitreous, which is opposed to the retina, forms a membrane on the surface of the retina.

The vitreous is firmly attached at two rings in the eye—one around the optic nerve and one as a band around the front edge of the retina where the retina joins the back edge of the ciliary body. The tightest attachment is at the anterior band. Everywhere else the back surface lies against the retina and is not attached firmly, except at scars and occasionally at blood vessels on the surface of the retina.

As the vitreous body shrinks, it pulls loose from the retina. If the vitreous is attached firmly to the retina in a spot, or a region, it pulls on the retina. This traction causes the photo elements of the retina, the rods and cones, to fire, sending a signal to the brain which the brain interprets as light. These impulses often occur in circles around the traction point, causing them to look like fireworks.

I have had many patients come to me because they saw, "a flash of light in the corner of my eye." They describe it as lighting or a crescent of light at the edge of their vision. They usually see it just after they turn out the light when they go to bed or after entering a darkened area. This phenomenon has come to be known as Moore's lightning streaks.

When the vitreous becomes completely detached from the retina, all the way up to the firm attachment ring in the front of the eye, it can pull on the circular attachment at the forward edge of the retina, causing the retina along that circle to respond with a light image. The shape of the attachment makes it a linear flash to the side of the person that is interpreted as lightning. This lightning appears in the temporal vision because the brain has shut off the temporal retinal area that corresponds to the view of the nose. A tug on the temporal retina would cause a nasal flash, if the retina was not suppressed in that area. These lightning flashes are usually considered harmless, but a good examination of the peripheral retina is warranted to rule out a tear or disinsertion of the edge of the retina when these streaks are first seen. Once the absence of tears is determined, they can be ignored.

If the traction causes the retina to tear, the nerves at the edge of the tear may fire off with flashes. The tear may cause capillary bleeding from the retina, either as a small clot or diffuse micro clots in the vitreous. These clots or scattered clumped blood cells cast shadows on the retina and appear as black spots. Since they are suspended in the vitreous, they can move around within the eye as the vitreous swirls with eye movement, like debris floating in water in a moving bucket. That is why they are called floaters.

When the vitreous pulls away from the attachment around the optic nerve, it is often opaque at the circle of attachment. This may appear as a circular floater or assume other shapes.

> A seventy-year-old lady came to see me saying that she had something floating in her vision that looked like a cockroach. She had called the exterminator three times complaining that their treatment of her house was not getting rid of the cockroaches. When she realized that the problem was in her eye, she wanted it removed. I explained that the procedure to remove it would probably make more floaters and might lead to retinal detachment or infection.
>
> Removing a speck of sugar from Jell-O will mess up the Jell-O more than the original speck. I explained to her that the brain often learns to ignore floaters and that as the vitreous shrank, the "cockroach" would be farther from the retina and become blurred and easier to ignore.

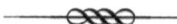

> Another older lady told me that she had a butterfly in her eye that flitted around. She liked it and said that it kept her company. She was sorry to lose it when it disappeared.

About one in ten people who have flashes and floaters have a tear in the retina that will develop into a retinal detachment if the tear is not treated immediately. For this reason, flashes and floaters are considered an ophthalmic emergency. Complaints of these symptoms demand a detailed ocular examination with evaluation of the entire retina through a dilated pupil as soon as it can be arranged. Nurses and receptionists in ophthalmologist's offices are trained to recognize these symptoms and respond with immediate access to the doctor, usually on the same day.

A tear in the retina can develop without signs of flashes or floaters, especially when they occur in the temporal retina. The brain has learned not to see with the far temporal retina because it always sees the side of the nose. That portion of the retina does not see and therefore does not flash. Slow development of a tear may not have sufficient hemorrhage to show as floaters. Therefore the retina may slowly detach and peel away from the underlying choroid, losing its posterior blood supply. As the retina detaches it loses the ability to see, creating a dark area in the vision corresponding to the area of the detachment. This is described by the patient as a curtain or shadow coming across the vision in the eye of the detachment. Good vision in the corresponding area of the other eye may fill in the picture in the brain and mask this dark area, delaying the patient's recognition of the shadow. The patient's description of the position of this curtain or shadow can lead the doctor to the area of detachment.

Most retinal detachments are caused by holes in the retina.

Sometimes there is more than one hole. Many holes occur in the temporal retina. Often, a person with a detachment in one eye will have a hole in the other eye which has not progressed to a detachment. The treatment of holes is usually done by burning the retina around the hole with a laser to "spot weld" the retina to the choroid to seal the hole. The inflammation, caused by the laser, produces scarring that binds the retina and choroid together. Once the retina has detached around the hole and becomes elevated, the laser will not seal it to the choroid unless it is first approximated to the choroid.

Treatment of a retinal detachment requires closing of the hole that caused it. If there is more than one hole, all holes must be closed. The retina in the eye is like the inner tube of a tire. If it is intact, inflating the inner tube pushes it against the wall of the tire. If there is a hole in the inner tube, air leaks out relieving the pressure and the inner tube can collapse away from the tire wall.

The hole in the retina allows the fluid in the eye to leak through the hole and peel the retina away from the eye wall and choroid.

If the holes are all closed, the choroid will remove the fluid that has collected between these two structures.

Once the retina has detached, there are several ways to make it reattach. Early repair is necessary to avoid progression to the central retina and central vision. Once the macula has detached, the vision may not return completely in the detached area after it has been put back in position.

When I trained, the retina and choroid were brought together by putting a band around the eye to cinch the sclera and choroid down to the detached retina and the fluid was drained from the space beneath the retina to allow the retina to drape over the buckled choroid. The choroid was frozen, thawed, and refrozen with a cryoprobe to cause inflammation that will glue the retina and choroid together to seal the holes. Sometimes a synthetic sponge was sutured to the outside of the eyeball to fold in the sclera and choroid more deeply against the retina.

Fifty years ago, some retinal surgeons used a tiny tack to hold the retina against the choroid. These were difficult to place and did not work very well. Newer techniques have been developed which work much better.

Dr. Freeman in Boston developed a technique of injecting an air bubble into the eye to push the retina against the buckled choroid until it healed. He had a special operating table which would spin, end over end, to position the bubble and lift the retina.

He would often sit on the floor, looking up at the eye of the patient who was suspended above him as he operated. The air was absorbed and disappeared after three to five days, often before healing was complete. Bubbles were injected again into the eyes.

Doctors began using other gasses, like sulfur hexafluoride (SF6), that were slower to absorb and lasted for seven to ten days, allowing longer time to heal and seal the retinal holes.

This bubble technique is now used without buckling surgery, in small detachments, to push the retina against the freeze treated choroid. This can be an office procedure, avoiding expensive hospitalization, if the hole is in a good location. The bubble must lift the retina against the choroid. To accomplish this approximation, sometimes the patient must lie on their side or sit up all the time to position the bubble against the retina. A Striker Frame bed can be turned 360 degrees to reposition the bubble and place the patient face down or head down to put the bubble where it needs to be. Another type of frame sandwiches the patient between front and rear frames so that they can be rotated around the body axis to position the bubble from side to side with the patient ending up face down.

My stock broker called me in the evening a few weeks ago to ask if flashes of light and lots of new black spots meant anything. This was several weeks after her cataract surgery.

She had undergone cataract surgery by a prominent local ophthalmologist and had reported very blurred vision the next day. Her ophthalmologist told her, on her first post op visit, that the capsule of her lens had torn and a small part of her cataract had fallen into the back of her eye.

He sent her the next day to see a retina specialist who scheduled immediate vitrectomy surgery (removal of the vitreous) to remove the fallen lens particle. Everything went smoothly and her vision improved over the next few weeks. She had undergone cataract surgery on her second eye the next week. (I had advised her to wait longer, but she went with her surgeon's advice.) Now she had developed flashes and floaters in the first eye that was operated for the dropped lens fragment. She told me that she was scheduled to see the retina surgeon again the next morning.

I told her to have him check for a retinal detachment in the first operated eye.

She called me again about a week later to tell me that the retinal surgeon had found a small retinal detachment and had put a bubble in her eye that day. Now her retina was attached and she was doing well, but her vision in that eye was not as good as it was in the second cataract surgery eye and she still had lots of floaters. After several more weeks the floaters went away and her vision was good in both eyes.

Shortly after I moved to Pennsylvania, a partially retired ophthalmologist called to ask me to see a seventy-five-year-old patient of his who was seeing new floaters. He was very near sighted so he was in a high risk group for retinal detachment. A complete eye exam showed that he did not have any holes or tears to explain his floaters.

Several months later he called to say that he was seeing a wisp of smoke swirling in his vision. Bleeding may present as a spiral stream of dispersing blood, a streak, or a blob.

I saw him within two hours of his call and saw scattered blood cells in his vitreous, but I could not find a clot or tear to show me the source of the blood. As I was explaining my findings to the patient, his wife spoke up to remind him to ask a question.

He blushed as he told me that he and his wife were enjoying sexual intercourse when he first noticed the swirling smoke. He wanted to know if that activity had caused his hemorrhage. I told him that I had recently heard a presentation by Dr. Thomas Friberg, a retina specialist. He reported several patients with intraocular hemorrhages during sex. Patients in that study did not have repeat hemorrhages.

I warned my patient that retinal hemorrhages do occur after trauma and other violent movements. He interrupted me to say that what they really wanted to know was whether there were any positions they should avoid. That subject was not covered in the presentation so I advised moderation. He did not have recurrences during the three more years that I followed his eye problems.

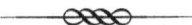

A forty-five-year-old man came to the clinic with a large shadow that seemed to him to be growing from his nose.

His retina was detached in the superior temporal area with a hole near the attachment of the vitreous. We called in the retinal surgeon who did a surgical buckle and attached the retina. He was in the hospital for about a week after the surgery. When we made rounds on about the third day, he asked if the headache that he had the night before his retinal detachment had caused it.

We explained that retinal detachments are painless and his headache would not have caused the retina to detach.

We told him that detachments occurred spontaneously or because of trauma to the eye such as being hit by a tennis ball or vigorously rubbing the eye. Then, he asked if the hospital had massage vibrators. When I asked him why he wanted a massage vibrator, he said that he had a vibrating massage device at home. He held it to his temple and forehead when he got a headache. He had used his vibrator at home to treat his headache the night before he came in. We decided that a vibrator, on or near his eye, could have shaken his eye to make or enlarge a retinal hole and thereby caused his detachment. I learned that a headache could have, indirectly, caused his detachment if he treated it with a vibrator around his eye.

When there are hemorrhages into the vitreous, they often disperse and clear completely. If there is sufficient blood, the hemorrhage may organize into a scar, or membrane, within the vitreous.

Diabetics with recurrent vitreous hemorrhages may form several membranes that are dense enough to block vision to the extent that the eye can only see very bright light, but no forms. Since these membranes were attached to the retina, they could not be removed without risk of tearing the retina. In the early nineteen seventies, several instruments were designed that enabled ocular surgeons to nibble holes in these membranes to restore vision without tearing the retina.

A sixty-four-year-old refinery worker came to see me in 1976, saying that he had lost all useful vision in his right eye as a child. He had recently developed a "curtain" in his good eye that bothered him when he drove his car.

This curtain hung down in front of his vision and swept back and forth in his good eye. If he jerked his eye to one side, the curtain would swing out of the way and his vision cleared. After a few seconds the curtain would settle back in front of his vision. When he would lie on his back in bed, the curtain went away allowing him to see the ceiling fan clearly.

His vitreous had detached from the retina in his good eye. On the back of the vitreous was a fibrous membrane, from some prior inflammatory episode of the upper retina.

When it hung down from its attachment in the top front of the eye, it partially blocked the light from reaching his retina. Before it peeled loose, it had been against the upper retina near the front of the eye where it did not interfere with his vision. Now, when his eye moved, the membrane swung around from the firm attachment on the upper retina. It swirled like the snow in a Christmas glass ball. Once the vitreous in the eye stopped moving, the membrane hung down behind the lens, blocking his vision. When he would lie on his back and look up, the membrane would hang back toward the top of the eye, out of the way.

We removed the membrane and the rest of his vitreous surgically, so that he could see. By removing the vitreous gel, there was nothing to which fibrosis could attach, so the membrane could not recur.

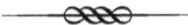

An ophthalmologist sent me a patient shortly after we had obtained our vitrectomy instrument. A sixteen-year-old boy, on his high school swim team, had been swimming in the high school pool when he collided with another swimmer. He was struck in the eye by the hand of the other swimmer and had a severe hemorrhage in his eye.

The referring doctor said that the boy had blood in the front of the eye which took several weeks to clear. By the time the ophthalmologist could see into the eye, the boy had developed a cataract from the trauma. The cataract was not dense, but he could not see the retina. This led him to believe that there had been hemorrhage into the vitreous also. He sent the boy to us to manage, because he did not have the ability to manage vitreous hemorrhage.

We performed an ultrasound examination of the eye and determined that the retina was not detached, but there was a lot of echo noise from the vitreous, indicating that there was probably blood diffusely throughout the vitreous gel. His cataract had become so dense by the time we saw him that we could not see the vitreous behind the cataractous lens.

I used the vitrectomy instrument to remove his cataract and discovered that the vitreous was not clear, but resembled cotton candy. The vitrectomy instrument was able to nibble the hazy vitreous to remove it from the eye.

When most of the vitreous was removed, I could see the retina through the haze and carefully peeled the vitreous gel from the surface of the retina and nibbled the resulting membrane of cloudy vitreous. The retina appeared completely normal and I could not identify the source of the bleeding. The bleeding site was probably from the ciliary body at the site of the trauma which I could not see. A fringe of the cloudy vitreous was left where it attached to the front edge of the retina to avoid causing a retinal tear and detachment.

The day following surgery, I held a pinhole and a plus 10 Diopter lens in front of his eye to compensate for the power of the cataractous lens I had removed. This allowed him to read at the 20/40 level. Over the next few days he could read 20/20 with a prescription spectacle lens.

Because the new spectacle lens was outside of the eye, rather than in the position of the cataract that it replaced, it would magnify the image in that eye. In order to use both eyes together, he would be fit with a contact lens which would magnify the image less, allowing him to see with both eyes and create depth perception vision for him.

We had to wait several weeks to fit the contact lens.

When I sent him home, several days after the surgery, he asked me if he could go back to work as a busboy. He was one of five children and worked part time as a busboy after school to help his family pay their bills. I told him he could go back to work, but he should not fill the bussing pans very full and take more trips to the kitchen. God bless him! He wanted to get back to work to help his family, rather than claim disability because of his eye.

At six weeks, I fit him for a contact lens with which he could see 20/20 and have good depth perception. It was very satisfying to be able to help this young man. I told him to wear goggles or remove the contact when he swam. The contact is held on the eye by the surface tension of the tears behind it. When the lens is surrounded by water, it can float free from the eye and is hard to find and retrieve from the swimming pool. His family could not afford many replacement lenses.

RAPID VISION LOSS

Sudden vision loss is usually an emergency. It may be partial dimming, segmental blurring, or complete loss of all light perception. The loss may be in one eye or both. These factors are often indicative of the cause of the visual loss.

Sudden loss of vision in one eye is usually vascular, occurring within or near the eye. Closure of the central retinal artery will cause total loss of vision in two or three minutes. After the artery enters the eye, it branches in to several arteries to supply parts of the retina. Branch retinal artery occlusion will cause a blind spot the size and shape of the portion of the retina supplied by the occluded branch. This blind spot is upside down and backwards from the location of the occluded branch artery. Artery occlusions within the eye usually occur in only one eye.

If the occlusion is not relieved within ten to twenty minutes, the vision will not return, even after the vessel is open again. The optic nerve and the retina are derived from the neural crest during embryonic development so they respond to lack of oxygen in the same way as the brain. Peripheral nerves will regenerate, following the neural sheath of the dead nerve and innervate the distribution of the dead nerve again. Brain does not regenerate so the optic nerve will not recover from a central retinal artery occlusion once the nerve dies from lack of oxygen.

The major causes of central retinal artery occlusion are high blood pressure and diabetes. Long standing hypertension (high blood pressure) will lead to arteriosclerosis, narrowing the vessels and increasing the chance of occlusion. After a retinal vein occlusion, all of these conditions should be looked for and treated by a physician, if present, to avoid occlusion of the other eye.

Atherosclerosis (cholesterol plaques on the artery walls) may cause artery occlusion by breaking free of the vessel wall to form an embolus that is carried by the blood until the embolus blocks the artery as the artery branches and narrows. The first branch of the carotid artery, after it enters the skull is the ophthalmic artery.

Small emboli may occlude the ophthalmic artery well behind the eye, damaging the optic nerve. The swelling caused by this blockage of oxygen (infarction) is far behind the eye and is not seen on the optic nerve within the eye. If the embolus reaches the end of the optic nerve where it enters the eye, the resulting swelling of the nerve protrudes into the eye and swells the head of the optic nerve. This is called papilledema. The swelling may spread into the nerve fiber layer on the surface of the retina wherever the blood supply is blocked. The macula is so thin that it does not become white from swelling (edema), but appears red in the center of the white swollen retina. This is described as a cherry red spot, the hallmark of central retinal artery obstruction.

If there is a cilio-retinal artery entering the eye at the temporal edge of the optic disc, it will supply the macula, sparing it from the damage of the central retinal artery occlusion. This artery arises from the ciliary arteries, not the central retinal artery, so it is not occluded when the central retinal artery is blocked.

The patient will have a narrow, horizontal slit of good vision that remains after the central retinal artery occlusion. About 14% of people have a cilio-retinal artery. Blockage of the cilio-retinal artery is very rare. When this does occur, it leaves a horizontal central blind spot in a full visual field. The blind spot extends from the optic nerve to the macula.

If the embolus is small, it may progress through the central ophthalmic artery and into one of the retinal artery branches. The artery usually divides into superior and inferior branches, each supplying half of the retina. These divide immediately into nasal and temporal branches which subdivide further as they spread to the peripheral retina.

Treatment of the central retinal artery occlusion is directed to moving the embolus from the central artery to one of the branches and then as far out onto the retina as possible to minimize the area of retina that is blocked of blood supply.

Breathing into and rebreathing from a small paper bag increases the carbon dioxide and lowers the oxygen accumulation in the blood, causing vascular dilation in the eye and throughout the body. Injection of a local anesthetic agent into the eye socket behind the eyeball will relax the eye muscles, lowering intraocular pressure which is the pressure on the outside of the blood vessels.

This allows the blood pressure to dilate the vessels. The anesthesia also dilates the retinal artery. This may allow the embolus to move down the artery to the peripheral retina.

To optimally lower the pressure in the eye, an ophthalmologist may insert a tiny needle into the front chamber of the eye to drain the fluid from there, lowering the pressure to room pressure.

The injection of the anesthetic and draining of ocular fluids must be done by a doctor, who has experience with these procedures, within the first twenty minutes to allow recovery. This return of vision depends on being at the right place at the right time. Care must be taken to avoid damaging the iris, cornea or lens with the needle. Sometimes, the anoxia caused by the occlusion of the vessel will cause the artery to dilate. This allows the embolus to spontaneously move further in the artery causing a smaller area of vision loss.

Patients come to the emergency room complaining that half of their vision went out suddenly, like a descending or ascending curtain that stopped at the horizontal midline. This is a branch retinal artery occlusion. These often resolve over the next several minutes as the embolus moves into the periphery. When this happens, we look for the embolus in the peripheral retina, but rarely find one.

The short duration of this episode leads us to call this a transient ischemic attack or TIA TIAs indicate the presence of atherosclerosis.

Some physicians will start Coumadin or other anticoagulant therapy to thin the blood to prevent further vascular plaques and allow the old plaques to stabilize or disappear. Some physicians will start the patient on daily aspirin for a lesser form of anticoagulant therapy.

The thin blood will not form plaques on the vessel walls as easily and may prevent recurrence of TIAs.

Occlusion of the central retinal vein that drains the blood from the retina will decrease vision and progress from haze and smokiness to very dim vision in about ten to fifteen minutes.

Branch retinal vein occlusion causes a relative blind spot, usually with some vision remaining, inversely proportional to the area of blocked drainage. Central vision often drops to the 20/400 level after central retinal vein occlusion. It may remain at that level for several days to weeks, but usually returns to usable central vision.

If the occlusion is permanent, the retinal veins will send new vessels to connect with open vessels and a secondary blood supply may be produced. In branch retinal vein occlusion that involves either the upper or lower half of the retina, new vessels from the open half will drain the other half. This may take several weeks to develop. Edema from the damaged retina may cause the macula to swell, decreasing central vision in the good half of the retina and the edge of adjacent retina, further decreasing central vision.

The damaged part of the retina in a branch vein occlusion may produce Vascular Endothelial Growth Factor called VEGF, a substance that encourages new vessel growth. This causes the new vessels to drain the occluded half of the retina, but it may cause neovascularization in unwanted places like around the optic nerve. Laser oblation of the damaged retina will reduce the amount of VEGF produced and should decrease the amount of neovascularization. The new treatments for macular degeneration, using anti-VEGF drugs, show some promise for treating this edema to restore better vision.

Certain medications are known to cause central retinal artery occlusion and sudden blindness. Two commonly used medication that do this are sildenafil (Viagra) and hydroxychloroquine (Plaquinil). The mechanism for this sudden blockage is unknown. Fortunately, this is a very rare side effect of these drugs.

People who have had a retinal artery occlusion should not take these medicines.

People with swelling of the optic nerve, called papilledema, have "transient obscurations of vision." or blackouts. Papilledema is caused by increased intracranial pressure—increased pressure inside of the skull. The optic nerve is enclosed in a membrane that is a continuation of the meninges that surround the brain.

Pressure within the skull is transmitted to this sheath around the optic nerve, blocking venous flow and causing the nerve head to swell into the eye. This usually does not affect vision, but may cause sudden blackouts of vision that last a few seconds. These blackouts are called transient obscurations. They are rare, but they are the only acute visual sign of papilledema. Increased intracranial pressure is caused by tumors of the brain, high blood pressure, head trauma, and a condition known as pseudotumor cerebrii.

Pseudotumor cerebrii occurs mostly in women of child bearing age. It is hormonally related which makes it most common during pregnancy or while taking birth control pills. It can be caused by medications like tetracycline and steroids. Removal of the cause is usually sufficient treatment, but idiopathic causes require diuretic medication and even lumbar puncture to relieve the pressure and resulting headaches.

Trauma to the front of the head, like in an auto accident with the head hitting the dashboard can cause the optic nerves to be pressed against the sharp edge of the bone surrounding back end of the optic canal where the nerve leaves the skull to pass through the optic canals to enter the eye socket. This can bruise the optic nerve (optic nerve contusion), causing slowly progressive blindness (10 to 30 minutes), or it can sever the nerve (optic nerve transection), causing sudden and permanent blindness.

Treatment of the bruised nerve is by controlling the swelling with medications like steroids, or by neurosurgically opening the optic canal to stop the pressure on the swollen nerve.

When the nerve swells in a bony canal it compresses the arteries and capillaries which nourish the nerve, damaging the nerve.

Immediately opening the optic canal (unroofing from the top through the skull) allows the nerve to expand which may keep the swollen nerve alive and allow vision to recover. This procedure will not help a severed optic nerve. The sudden or slow onset of blindness is the best clue to determine if the nerve is severed or only bruised. Concussion with loss of consciousness caused by the accident may obscure this discriminator.

VISION COLOR CHANGES

One form of vision color problem is color blindness. Color blindness can be hereditary or acquired. It can be manifested in several ways. Color vision happens in the cones in the retina. There is a set of cones for red and green colors and another set for yellow and blue vision. The most common form of color blindness is loss of discrimination of red and green. Loss of yellow and blue vision is less common. If both color sets are involved, color blind people may see only in black and white.

Color blindness occurs in about 7% of males and less than 1% of females. Color vision loss may be complete or partial which may allow the affected person to tell a red light from a green one, but they have trouble matching the colors of their clothes. Most color vision loss is genetic so it runs in families.

There is an instrument, called an anomaloscope that allows measurement of the relative loss of red and green color discrimination.

Since the mixture of red and green light in equal parts creates yellow light for a normal person, this machine mixes red and green light on a screen to form yellow light. The partially color blind person turns the dials on the apparatus to mix red and green light to match a pure sodium yellow light in an adjacent light panel. By using a standard green or red setting and using the other light color to match the yellow, the amount of red suppression or green suppression can be measured.

There are special cards, called Hary Rand Rittler (HRR) or Ishihara plates that are used to detect color vision loss. These cards show a field of dots that are printed in the same brightness density using different colors. A color blind person cannot tell the dots apart because of the matching color density. The colors of the dots are arranged to make letters or numbers. A person with color blindness cannot see the difference in the color of the dots so they do not see the figures. The cards are made to show red-green or yellow-blue loss.

Other forms of color vision tests include a 100 hue test wherein the person is asked to arrange 80 color dots (chosen from 100 hues) in order, from blue to red, in the spectrum. The dots are numbered on the bottom so the tester can determine how far they are out of order. The pattern of errors is charted on a circular diagram to determine whether the defect is red-green or yellow-blue.

There is also a yarn sorters test in which a bundle of closely colored yarn strands are presented. The person is asked to separate the yarns into smaller bundles of exactly the same color.

This test is used to select workers in textile factories who have to match different dye lots.

> When I practiced in Texas, The Maritime Academy of Texas A & M University would send two or three students each year for color vision testing. Maritime certification requires that the person with maritime papers have good color vision. The channel markers are in red and green. The rule is "Red on the Right, Returning to port." Red markers are kept to the right of the ship and green markers are kept to the left with the channel in between. A sea pilot who cannot tell red from green may soon run a ship aground.
>
> These students who failed the color vision testing, would plead with us to try other tests to show that they

had some color vision so they could stay in school to become merchant marine officers.

There are contact lenses with a pink tint that allow color blind individuals to tell red from green, but these are not allowed for these sea captains. They do help in driving, helping to see stop lights. In recent years, the lenses of traffic lights have been made red-orange and blue-green to allow people who are red-green blind but still have yellow-blue vision to tell apart the color of stoplights. This works well for those who are red-green only in color deficiency. Vertical stoplights almost always have the red on top and green on the bottom, but horizontal stoplights can be confusing.

> The little town of Mountain Home, Arkansas, near my parent's retirement home, had stoplights that had the red lenses on top for east and west and the red lenses on the bottom for north and south. They were opposite for the green lenses. All four directions of the middle lenses were yellow. The single light bulb at each level, located in the middle of the column illuminated all four directions at once. This was very economical, but confusing to color blind people. I never learned if this was a cause of traffic accidents in Mountain Home.

Color vision changes can be caused by certain medications.

People taking digitalis for heart conditions may notice a yellow tint to everything when they have taken too much digitalis and are considered digitalis toxic. Decreasing the dose will allow the colors to return to normal.

ViagraR has been shown to cause a blue tint to everything for some people. This tint goes away when the Viagra wears off.

Viagra has also been reported to cause sudden irreversible vision loss, usually in only one eye at a time. This is a rare event which should cause the affected person to stop the use of Viagra immediately so that blindness does not happen in the second eye. This side effect is thought to occur in men who have a predisposition to central retinal artery closure, such as hypertension, diabetes, or atherosclerosis.

People who report that everything has a red or pink tint probably have a hemorrhage in the eye which has diffused throughout the vitreous jelly that fills the eye. If the hemorrhage is small, it will probably clear and colors will return to normal. The person should seek an eye exam to find the cause of the hemorrhage so that it can be treated.

Toxicity of the retina to certain drugs such as Plaquinil can be detected early by testing for loss of peripheral vision to red light or by color vision testing. This is done every few months when following patients on Plaquinil (hydroxychloroquine) to see if they are becoming toxic.

Part II

DISEASES OF ALL AGES

REFRACTIVE DISORDERS: MYOPIA, HYPEROPIA, ASTIGMATISM AND PRESBYOPIA

The eye is a unique organ that focuses the light as it enters through the cornea, passes through the pupil and the lens and shines on the retina. Light rays, reflecting from an object, radiate in all directions from the object. From a specific point on a distant object, the rays of light that are close enough together to enter the pupil of the eye are essentially parallel. The curve of the cornea and the optical power of the human lens bend the essentially parallel rays of light to converge them to a point.

The cornea and the crystalline lens both converge the light rays to bring them to a single point. The point where rays converge to form a spot should be on, or close to, the retina. The points of the image projected on the retina by this focusing mechanism are upside down and reversed, right to left. That is, the light entering the eye from the right side is focused on the left side of the retina. Light from the left will be focused on the right side of the retina. The same is true for above and below. Looking through a pin hole excludes the other parallel rays so that only a few of the straight rays pass through the hole and therefore do not need to be focused. This is how a pinhole camera works. The pupil is larger than a pin hole so the light must be focused to get a clear picture on the retina. The brain turns the image right side up and corrects the right to left reversal.

If all eyes were perfectly shaped, everyone would be able to see without glasses, a condition known as emmetropia. This could exist until they reached the age when the lens becomes stiff and does not focus on near objects. Unfortunately, some eyes are longer or shorter than they should be for perfect focus. Or the cornea may bend light more or less than normal making the eye out of focus. If the lens has been removed, because it became a cataract or was damaged, the eye will be very farsighted, focused out past the moon.

Visual acuity

Vision is measured in several ways. The most common is by using a standardized chart of letters, numbers, or line figures at a fixed distance. The standard distance of the patient from the chart is twenty feet for distance and fourteen inches for near. Most doctors' offices are not twenty feet long, so mirrors are used to give the twenty foot total distance. The height of the letters that can be seen any distance must span an arc of five minutes on the retina. The smallest letter that can be seen by an average person at twenty feet will project on the retina as the same size, five minutes or arc, as one that is ten times larger, but at two hundred feet away. The letter at one hundred feet would be five times larger than the one at twenty feet.

When the various letters for different distances are placed on the same chart at twenty feet away, the patient can read at twenty feet, what a normal person can see at the given distance for that letter. The vision of 20/20 is normal. A result of 20/100 would mean that the patient can only see letters at twenty feet that a normal person can see at one hundred feet away. When a person can only see the 20/200 letter or larger at twenty feet with the better eye, they are considered legally blind and can check that box on their tax return. A small percentage of people can see letters that are smaller than the 20/20 letters. There is a 20/15 line and a 20/10 line on most eye charts.

> I did an examination on a Navy pilot for the renewal of his flying license. He read the 20/15 line perfectly, so I reported that on the examination record. The Navy sent it back to me saying that the best anyone could see was 20/20 so my measurement of 20/15 was incorrect. I knew better, but changed the form so the pilot could get his license. When I was younger, I could read the 20/10 line from twenty feet.

When the person cannot see any of the letters on the chart at twenty feet we decrease the distance to the chart until they can see the 20/200 letter. If they see it at ten feet, it is recorded as 10/200. This would be the same as 20/400.

Charts with the letter E facing in different directions or line drawings of familiar objects (teddy bear, birthday cake, etc.), or numbers can be used for children and illiterate adults.

If they cannot see the 20/200 letter at five feet, 5/200, we ask them to count the number of fingers that the examiner holds in front of their eye at about three feet away. The fingers are brought closer to the patient until they can accurately count them. In reality, one, two and four fingers are easier to count than three so we use those fingers. The vision is recorded as count fingers at that distance, C.F. @ 1 foot for example.

If the person still cannot count fingers at six inches, the examiner asks the patient to say what direction his hand is moving as they wave it in front of the patient's eye. The examiner must be careful not to touch the patient with their other hand while they are doing this, because that might betray which way they are moving the testing hand. (Have the patient cover his other eye with he palm of his own hand.) If they can identify the motion, it is recorded as H.M. vision.

> I had a ninety-six-year-old patient who could not see my hand moving, but he insisted that he could tell me which way his own hand was moving in front of his eye. That, of course, did not count.

In the situation where the patient cannot see hand movements, a bright light, such as a fresh pen light, is shown into the eye. If the patient says that they can see it, they are asked to tell when it is off and on while the examiner turns the light off and on. This must be done in a noiseless manner to avoid giving the person clues. The light can be moved toward and away from the pupil while it is on. If the patient can see the light, different colored lights are used to see if they can discriminate colors. I used the different colored bottle caps from the eye drop bottles placed over the pen light. This is a higher level function for the retina that just white light. Then the light is directed through the pupil at the right, left, upper and lower retina so see if the patient can determine the direction from which the light is coming (called projection). This is recorded as L.P. with or without projection and with or without color. With a very dense cataract or dense diabetic vitreous membranes, these variations are very critical in deciding whether surgical intervention might be successful.

It is very discouraging to undergo surgery and then not see a difference in the outcome. I operated on many diabetics with light perception and projection and color discrimination who were able to see 20/40 or better after the diabetic membranes were removed from their eye.

There are vision charts or cards for near vision, usually printed with numbers or tumbling E's. The sizes are calibrated as near 20/20, 20/40, etc. or called by Jaeger numbers such as J1 or J5. J1+ is 20/20, J2 is 20/30, J10 is 20/100, etc. These cards are used for fitting bifocals or other near vision glasses and for vision checks when a wall chart is not available. People over forty-five years old should wear reading glasses or bifocals when reading these near cards.

The area of vision is also measured. It is called the visual field.

It measures how far off center of vision that the eye can perceive a spot or light, either moving (dynamic) or in one place (static) with the eye looking straight ahead. When measuring a visual field on a patient with either glaucoma or a neurological problem, the field is checked in multiple meridians throughout 360 degrees from the center of vision. The pattern of the area of missing vision is often helpful in determining the location of the problem in the eye, optic nerve, optic tracts or brain cortex.

To drive a car in most states, the width of the visual field for a one centimeter white spot against a black background, with both eyes open, must total one hundred degrees in the horizontal direction. A person with less than twenty degrees of vision from side to side in the better eye is considered legally blind.

When the patient may have had a stroke or a brain tumor, it is important to know if they can see in all four quadrants of the visual field with each eye. For a screening examination, the person is asked to count the number of fingers held in each quadrant.

For more subtle loss, the person is asked to use both eyes and total the number of fingers held with both in hands in different quadrants simultaneously. If a defect is suspected, a formal visual field test for each eye may determine the location and nature of the problem.

There are other ways to check vision in children, trained animals, and busy astronauts, but I will not discuss them in this book.

Myopia

Myopia is when vision is better at near that at distance, often called near sightedness. When the eye focuses the light in front of the retina, not on the retina, because the cornea bends the rays too much or the eye was stretched too long, the eye is myopic, or nearsighted. To bring this eye into focus, the rays must be diverged (actually, less converged) so that the point of focus is on the retina. When the rays meet or focus in front of the retina, they cross and are diverging when they hit the retina. Instead of a point of light on the retina, they cast a blur circle. When the many points of an image become overlapping blur circles, the image is blurred and fine detail is lost.

How do you know if you are myopic? Most children do not complain about not being able to see distant things. They do not know that they should see them clearly. Infants and small children are concerned with things that are close to them. Many of my young patients told their parents, after they got their first pair of glasses, that they did not realize that they were supposed to be able to see the individual leaves on trees or the cracks in the sidewalk, etc.

To correct the focus of a myopic eye we can fit spectacles with diverging lenses (minus lenses) or a contact lens with minus power. When you look through this lens, things appear smaller.

The spectacle lens to correct large amounts of near sightedness makes the smaller letters on the vision chart too small to see.

Contact lenses do this to a lesser degree. People with very high myopia (-15 to -20D) cannot see the lower lines of the vision chart well enough to pass the test for a driver's license, because the glasses or contact lenses make the letters smaller.

The ophthalmologist or optometrist can determine the power of lens which correctly focuses the light on the retina, even in small children, by using a device called a retinoscope and a set of lenses. When these lenses are mounted in a series of wheels to suspend in front of the face, the apparatus is called a phoropter.

When a lens causes the movement of the retinoscope light beam to stop moving in the eye, that lens, when adjusted for working distance, will correct the vision in that eye. We can measure babies under anesthesia, non verbal patients and uncooperative patients that way.

We know that myopia is made worse by darkness. When we order sun glasses we often order an extra quarter Diopter of minus lens power in the prescription to counteract the effect of the decreased light (darkness) caused by the light dimming of the sun glasses.

Most people with myopia have elongated eyeballs. This stretches the retina and choroid making the retina thin and susceptible to forming holes. Therefore, people with high degrees of myopia are more prone to develop retinal detachments.

Hyperopia

The farsighted, or hyperopic, eye, is either shorter than the focus point of the cornea and lens, or the cornea is too flat and will not bend the light enough to focus it on the retina. In farsightedness, the light is actually focused behind the retina. The light has not become focused to a point so it creates a blur circle. To make it an image of points of light, we must fit spectacles or a contact lens to converge the light more, using a plus lens. Looking through a plus lens makes things larger and blurred, unless you are farsighted.

Fortunately, the lens of the eye can change shape to bend the light more, zooming in. This will correct small to moderate amounts of hyperopia, without glasses, in people younger than forty-five.

How do you know if you are hyperopic? Most hyperopic people do not know they are farsighted until they reach the age of presbyopia, the age when you have to hold things farther away to be able to see them clearly. People with hyperopia can focus in from their far point, (the distance that the eye is normally focused). When they direct their attention to an object that is closer than this natural focal distance, or far point, the brain automatically focuses the eye on that object. The object appears sharply focused.

People with hyperopia and astigmatism will have blurring from the astigmatism that is not corrected by the focusing.

When glasses or contacts are needed to correct the astigmatism, we will often correct part of the hyperopia when we correct the astigmatism, decreasing the amount of focusing the person must do to see clearly.

Suddenly correcting all of a patient's hyperopia requires several weeks of adaptation by the patient. People who are farsighted will focus away some of the hyperopia all of the time. When the hyperopia is corrected fully with glasses, the eye continues to do this habitual focusing which overcorrects the problem, making everything out of focus. For most people it takes about three weeks for the eye to relax the habitual focusing completely. To avoid this problem in adults, we only correct the amount that the patient accepts when the habitual focusing is not disabled by eye drops.

People with hyperopia usually have smaller eyes. This decrease from the size of a normal eye tends to crowd the structures in the front of the eye and may cause other problems such as narrow angle glaucoma. Since people with hyperopia usually see well without glasses, they tend to skip routine eye examinations. This means that they do not get the intraocular pressure checked, so glaucoma may be missed until it is very advanced. The routine exam, every two years, usually checks for things like intraocular tumors, diabetes, high blood pressure, glaucoma, and the many other diseases that can affect the eye.

A child that is born with a high degree of hyperopia may develop crossed eyes because focusing the eyes causes them to turn in toward the nose. This will be discussed in Chapter 31 on acquired eye problems in children, under strabismus.

Astigmatism

The cornea is not always a symmetrical sphere, so the amount of light bending for rays displaced horizontally may not be the same as for rays displaced vertically. One pair will be bent more that the other so both cannot be in focus on the retina. This is called astigmatism. Fortunately the cornea tends to warp or fold around a line or an axis. It is possible for the eye to be nearsighted in one meridian and farsighted in the meridian rotated ninety degrees away. When there is astigmatism, all meridians are usually either myopic or they are hyperopic, but to varying amounts.

How do you know if you have astigmatism? Since astigmatism is caused by warping of the cornea, vision will be distorted at all distances. Because this distortion is present all of the time, the patient may not know that things are distorted. Distortion is most obvious when reading print or looking at fixed patterns or objects like door frames, cabinets, etc. Distortion causes difficulty reading random letters, like on the vision testing chart. P's become R's or F's. (There are no Rs on the standard eye chart, but many people see them there.) The letters O, Q, and C are confused with one another. Most people learn that they have astigmatism when they are examined to determine the cause of blurred vision.

Hard contact lenses have a spherical front surface that bends the light. The tears fill in behind the lens obliterating the difference in curvatures, so hard contacts become a new front surface for the eyes and will correct astigmatism in most cases. Soft contact lenses conform to the eye, duplicating the warping of the cornea and therefore do not correct astigmatism well. New designs of soft lenses called toric lenses, can correct limited amounts of astigmatism.

The lens in the eye can focus inward from its usual focus point, but it cannot focus further away than its natural focus point. People who are farsighted are theoretically focused past infinity and can zoom in to see clearly at the desired distance.

Nearsighted people have eyes that focus at near with everything past that point being relatively blurred. They cannot zoom out.

Once they are corrected for distant focus with minus lenses, they can focus in with their own natural lens to see nearer objects.

Presbyopia

As the lens ages, it loses its flexibility and is unable to focus to a very near object. With time this near point moves further and further away and one must hold a book farther away to be able to focus on the print. This is known as presbyopia (old eyes). It usually occurs at about age forty-five, give or take five years. Since hyperopic people use some of their focusing to see at distance and need more to see at near, they may become presbyopic a few years earlier. This is often when they learn that they are hyperopic.

Presbyopia is treated with bifocals, trifocals, and progressive glasses, or with reading glasses. If the patient needs glasses to see at distance, they will need a different power of glasses to see at near. These two powers can both be ground into the same pair of glasses. Bifocals put the distance correction at the top of the lens and the near correction at the bottom. The person looks straight ahead, through the top, to see far away and down, through the near segment, called the add, to read, sew, or do other close work.

There are different shapes to the bifocal add part of the lens.

If the near part goes all of the way across the lens, it is called an executive lens. This type of lens works well for people who work at desks and need to see the whole top of the desk clearly. When the person is myopic, the add segment is round on the bottom with a flat top or straight top dividing near and far. Far sighted people need a near add which is round on top. This difference in shape is dictated by the way an image will jump when seen through the top and then the bottom of the lens.

> The first person I fit with bifocals was illiterate. He could not read the letters on the eye chart. He was an oyster shucker on the Chesapeake Bay. He had to see the crack between the shells of the oyster he was opening, but he had to watch for oyster boats to help them dock and then help unload them. He needed bifocals.

When I was in the Sahara Desert in Morocco, we came upon a nomadic family living in a large tent. An older woman was spinning wool into thread using a stick that she spun by hand. She was squinting her eyes to see the thread. I gave her a pair of Dollar Store reading glasees with +2.50 lenses. She put them on and looked at her yarn.

She looked up at me with a big smile. She could see her yarn much better. That evening a young man walked into our tent camp and asked one of our guides to speak to the man with the majic glasses. He had walked five miles across the desert to get a pair of the glasses for his mother who had heard about the glasses I had given to the other lady. Fortunately I had another pair to give to him.

Some people have trouble getting used to looking up to see at distance and looking down to see things at near. One way to learn this is to take an automobile trip and be the driver. To see the road, you must look up; to see the instrument panel you must look down. Most drivers to not move their head to do this, but they move their eyes up and down. Looking down at steps is a problem since the near segment of the glasses make the steps blurred. Usually the brain will move the feet the right amount by looking to the steps that are further away, up or down the steps. Looking down with the head to look through the top of the lenses helps with curbs and short sets of steps.

Many people need a clear focus for distances that are between across the room and reading distances. People who work at a desk or a work bench often need clear focus at twenty to thirty inches. This requires a third lens between the far and near lens, called a trifocal. Once computer lens grinding came into being, it was possible to design a program that ground a bulge onto the lens which contained curves that increased the power gradually and continually so that, at least in theory, all distances could be in focus, depending the part of the lens looked through. This is called a progressive lens or varifocal lens.

>An anesthesiologist came to me in Galveston, complaining that he could not read the fine print on medication ampoules. I started to fit him with bifocals, but I decided to explain progressive lenses to him. He jumped at the idea because he had so many visual demands at different distances in the operating room. He needed to see the charts and X-rays on the wall, the surgical site, the dials on his machine, and the fine print on the medication labels. He was very happy with his progressive lenses.

Shortly after my success with the anesthesiologist, a surgeon came to see me because he could not see what he was doing up close. He could see the X-rays on the light box on the wall, but he could not see what he was operating on in the abdomen. He had to wear his surgical magnifying glasses all of the time and they limited the area he could see at any one time. I fit him with progressive lenses. He told me over and over how much he liked them.

After about two years he came back wanting more power in the near lens. This was normal progression of presbyopia so I ordered stronger progressive lenses. He was back in a week complaining of the distortion caused by the progressive lenses. The optician said that he had changed suppliers for progressive lenses since the first pair had been made. He ordered the new power from the original supplier, but the doctor was still bothered by the distortion. He went through all four companies that made progressive lenses at that time, but he could not get over the distortion. I eventually had to put him in trifocals to satisfy his needs.

When I first tried progressive lenses it took about three weeks until I no longer could notice the distortion. My brain had adjusted to it and things did not look distorted anymore. Until then, my desk looked like there was a moving bump in the middle. The bump went away.

Another popular way to treat presbyopia is called mono-fit lenses. For people who do not need glasses for distance or they wear contact lenses for distance vision, one eye can be fit with a contact lens for near vision while the other eye sees at distance.

For people already wearing contacts, one contact is changed to see at near. The trick is to fit the dominant eye for distance and the non-dominant eye for near. Doing it the other way around drives people crazy. Most people cannot tolerate the dominant eye set for reading. People who are successful with the contact lens mono-fit will do well with cataract surgery where the implant lens power is set for near in the non-dominant eye. The rule is *Distance Dominant, Near Non-dominant*. The new generation of intraocular lenses may be able to focus in and out, creating a focusing condition for cataract a surgery patient that is similar to what it was before presbyopia created the need for reading glasses.

For people who do not need glasses for distance, simple reading glasses correct their reading problem very well. We like to give people only the amount of extra power they need to read comfortably. We start newly acquired presbyopia with +1.00 or +1.50 reading glasses. To remove all need to focus at normal reading distance of fourteen inches, mathematically would require a +2.50 lens. A person with presbyopia will need this full power at about four to six years after first noticing presbyopia. Meanwhile we go from +1.00 to +1.50 to +2.00 and then +2.50 in one to two year steps. Starting at +2.50 will make the person totally dependent on reading glasses almost immediately.

People, who do not wear glasses for distance, often like to use half glasses. These have only the bottom half a lens which is ground for near. The top of the lens is missing. The lens is mounted low so the person can look over the top to see at distance.

Some people feel that these glasses are intimidating. They are a favorite of professors and lawyers.

Reading glasses should be custom made by an optical shop if the right and left eye require different powers of spectacles for distance or if there is significant astigmatism. If there is little or no astigmatism and the eyes are the same amount of myopia or hyperopia, reading glasses can be bought at the drug store, dollar store or on line for as little as $6:00. I recommend taking a piece of the want ads with you to the store and trying to read the ads with different powers, from +1.00 to +2.50. Get that lowest power that allows you to read the fine print easily when it is held at about ten inches from the face. This will allow prolonged reading with out fatigue at the usual fourteen inch reading distance.

> I had a wealthy patient in Galveston who had undergone cataract surgery in both eyes with intraocular lens implants. He had an excellent result and saw 20/20 with both eyes at distance. He complained that he could not see to read the paper. Except for some new, still somewhat experimental intraocular lenses, implant lenses do not change focus. I put some +2.50 lenses in a trial frame and put them on him. I gave him the near card with examples of very fine print on it. He read the smallest print with ease. He immediately asked me to order these in glasses.
>
> I explained to him that "dime store" glasses would work for him and suggested that he buy pair of +2.50 readers at a dime store or drug store and try them. After cataract surgery, the full +2.50 power is needed to focus at near.

When he returned several weeks later, he told me that the drug store readers worked very well, so he had bought several pairs of readers. He had one in kitchen where he read the morning paper, one on his desk at work, one next to his easy chair in the living room, one in his airplane, one on his yacht, and one in his car. He had his wife carry an extra pair in her purse in case they were out somewhere like a restaurant. He bragged to me that he still had not spent as much as the custom made readers would have cost him. Thinking like that may be why he was so wealthy.

A fifty-five-year-old hematology technician who was the head of the leukemia laboratory came to me because she could not see at all of the distances she needed to see for her job and after work activities. She needed to look through the microscope which is optically set for long distance (no focusing). She also needed to put cover slips on slides at about five inches from her nose. She needed to reed bottles on the shelf at fifteen to twenty inches and supervise other people in the lab. She was also the church organist with music at about thirty inches away. She had worn contacts for years. She could look through the microscope while wearing her contacts. She had also worn half glasses for near for several years. This arrangement gave her one focus at distance and one at near. This was before progressive lenses.

I had the optician make her a pair of half glasses with a bifocal lens. The bottom lens was very strong for her to see clearly at five inches and the top was focused at fourteen inches (normal reading distance). She could see over the top of the half glasses for distance and the microscope. I had her buy a pair of reading half glasses at the drug store with a +1.50 or +2.00 lens so that she could read the music and see the choir director at the same time. She was very happy.

Bifocals are made in a special configuration for workers who must work over their heads, like electricians and carpenters.

There is an extra bifocal lens ground into the top of the lenses so that when they are looking up they can see at near for wiring or nailing.

A woman I was chatting with at a garden party recently asked me if it was normal for her to see double for several minutes after she had been reading. This was actually an example of under corrected myopia. She was about fifty years old and did not wear glasses. Her ophthalmologist had told her that she did not need glasses except for reading.

She had a pair of weak reading glasses which she used whenever she planned to read for a while. Because they were weak, she had to do some focusing to see at near.

She was still accommodating, or focusing, when she read.

Since her lens had become stiff from her age, it did not relax immediately when she stopped reading. This left her focused at near until the lens had relaxed and returned to its normal shape. She was temporarily myopic. I asked her if the double vision was side by side or vertically displaced.

She told me that it was vertically displaced, one above the other. I have had many under corrected myopic patients tell me that they saw double taillights, one above the other, when they drove at night. I do not know of an optical reason for this vertical double vision.

NEW WAYS TO CORRECT VISION WITHOUT GLASSES

Every girl has heard that, "Men never make passes at girls who wear glasses." Even though we know that this is not always true, many people do not like to wear glasses because they feel that they are unattractive. Although, I have known women who wear big dark glasses all the time, even indoors, because they feel they are glamorous. To avoid glasses, many people choose to wear contact lenses, especially since soft contact lenses are so comfortable. However, contact lenses are often a hassle with cleaning, soaking, inserting and removing. People want to see without glasses or contacts, so a lot of research has been done on ways to correct vision without glasses or contact lenses.

Contact lenses can be fit (or misfit) in such a way that they warp the cornea. By making the lens too steep or too flat, the cornea can be made more steep or flat to correct hyperopia or myopia. These lenses are usually worn at night to change the cornea shape. The changes may last for several days once the wearing is discontinued. The change in corneal curvature may correct the vision to 20/20 in some cases. This trick is often tried by men who want to qualify for flight school. Air force personnel must have 20/20 vision without glasses or contact lenses to qualify for flight school. Once they are in flight school, they can wear glasses or contacts.

This practice of shaping the cornea by wearing misfit contact lenses is called orthokeratology. The down side of this practice is that it may cause painful corneal epithelial defects or corneal ulcers that lead to scarring and permanent loss of vision. It tends to be very temporary, lasting only a few days.

> When I was in training, I wore hard contact lenses. I noticed that I was seeing about the same with, or without the lenses. I took them off at work on day and checked my vision on the vision chart. I read 20/20 without the contact lenses. I had been 20/40 without lenses when they were fit.
>
> I needed to change my driver's license to Massachusetts, so I went to the license office that afternoon and passed the vision test without glasses or contacts. Unfortunately, the corneal changes only lasted for two weeks, so I had to go back to the contact lenses.

Correcting vision without glasses or contact lenses requires changing the shape of the cornea or the eyeball. This requires surgery of some kind.

Radial keratotomy

The Japanese came up with the sharply curved Sato knife for making radial cuts in the back of the peripheral cornea. The blade was very small and curved and was sharp on the inside of the curve. It was inserted through a tiny stab wound at the edge of the cornea. The blade made a radial cut through the posterior two thirds of the cornea. This was repeated to make a circle of radial cuts in the back of the cornea. These cuts allowed the cornea to bulge forward around the edges and flatten in the center to treat myopia. This worked for a while, but the cuts in the back of the cornea damaged the endothelium, allowing it to leak ocular fluid into the corneal tissue and cause the cornea to become cloudy after several months.

The Russians, under Dr. Fyodorov, then made the radial cuts in the front surface of the edge of the cornea to avoid the endothelium. This procedure also allowed the outer part of the cornea to bulge slightly, flattening the center of the cornea making the focus point further back in the eye so light was focused on the retina without glasses. This was called radial keratotomy.

Doctors could make four, eight, or sixteen evenly spaced, deep, radial cuts in the cornea depending how much myopia was to be corrected. Unfortunately, the amount of surgery was difficult to predict so repeat surgeries were often needed. To make cuts of 90% of the corneal thickness in a repeatable manner, it was necessary to use a diamond blade with a micrometer set stop that limited the depth of the cut. Over corrections, leaving people far sighted, occurred too frequently. Fortunately, the eye can focus to overcome the resultant farsightedness, at least until the person becomes presbyopic in their forties. Then the over correction becomes manifest.

Lasers

Ophthalmology has always led the way with lasers and technology.

Lasers were being used in ophthalmology to treat diabetic retinopathy, glaucoma, and capsule opacities after cataract surgery.

A new laser became available that could vaporize tissue at a controlled rate. (In the TV show, Captain Video and the Video Rangers, they had the option to set their lasers either on stun or vaporize. This new laser was set on vaporize.)

Someone figured out that they could vaporize the front of the cornea to change its shape. By burning a spot in the center of the cornea and then enlarging the spot and burning a larger area, while burning the original spot again, and continuing to enlarge the spot, they could flatten the curve of the cornea with ever enlarging spots until the desired size and amount of flattening was reached.

The curve of the nearsighted cornea was measured and the measurements were fed into programs in a computer to determine the number of shots and the energy needed. The laser was programmed to fire automatically to obtain the desired corneal shape. This was called photo refractive keratectomy or PRK.

To get consistent results, the epithelial layer of cells had to be removed from the area of the cornea to be treated and then it had to grow back after the laser treatment. This caused significant pain for the first three or four days until the epithelium covered the treated area of the cornea. Laser surgeons did not want the post operative patients sitting in the waiting room with prospective laser patients, because the pain they were having scared off the potential laser patients.

The solution to this problem was to use a special knife, called a keratome, to shave off a thin layer of the cornea with the epithelium attached. Rather than shave this layer all the way off, the layer was left attached at one edge as the hinge of a flap. The flap was turned back and the laser vaporization was applied to the underlying cornea. After the cornea shape was changed by the laser, the flap, with the epithelium attached, was put back on the cornea. The cut epithelium edges healed rapidly, shortening the duration of the pain to a few hours. Some surgeons use a soft contact lens bandage to ease the pain on the first day. This procedure is called Lasik. There have been variations in flap design and laser programs to produce better results with fewer complications.

The new complications of Lasik were related to the flap. If the flap did not lay down smoothly on the underlying surface, wrinkles caused distortion. If the edges of the flap did not stick together immediately, the epithelium could grow between the cornea and the flap to cause optical distortion and a loose flap.

If there was debris on the cornea, such a dust or lint, when the flap was replaced, the foreign material was trapped under the flap. The trapped material could distort the corneal surface and interfere with light transmission through the cornea. If bacteria were trapped between the cornea and the flap, an infection could develop that would lead to scarring and distortion, even if it was treated successfully. There are a lot of "ifs," but fortunately they are rare. Surgeons rinse the surface of the cornea thoroughly before replacing the flap to avoid these complications.

Radial keratotomy and laser ablation for myopia were relatively simple, but the correction of hyperopia was more of a challenge.

Ablating the central cornea to flatten the cornea, for myopia, was straight forward. Causing the cornea to become steeper, by making a hump in the center of the cornea was a more complex problem. People tried to burn rings in the cornea to get it to contract in a circle to bulge the central cornea so that it would bend light more. Burning the cornea caused temporary results which lasted a few weeks. Laser sculpting to steepen the central cornea without thinning the peripheral cornea too much was difficult to program. New lasers that would dissolve the cornea from within have some promise, but laser correction of hyperopia has been more difficult to obtain.

There are limits to the amount of cornea that can be removed by laser to correct myopia. When the central cornea is too thin, the cornea bulges centrally, creating more myopia and a condition similar to keratoconus. Since keratoconus causes myopia, surgeons tried to treat the myopia of keratoconus patients with PRK. The laser made the central cornea thinner and allowed it to stretch and bulge more making vision worse and also making it harder to fit a contact lens to correct vision. Keratorefractive surgery with a knife or laser has its limits.

There are people who have much more myopia than a laser can correct (more than a power of about -8.00 D). Contact lenses have to be very thin in the middle and thick at the edge to get the power necessary to correct these people. This peripheral thickness, even with a tapered edge makes them hard to wear. The eyelid keeps knocking them off center or out of the eye.

Epikeratophakia

A procedure called epikeratophakia (surface cornea lens) was designed to help these people. A donor cornea is frozen to hardness and then cut with a lathe, the same way that contact lenses are made. This biological lens, with a wide, thin edge, is then freeze dried for storage. When a surgeon uses the lens it is rehydrated with saline to soften it before it is sewn onto the cornea.

The surgeon cuts a circular groove in the cornea with a trephine and undermines the outer edge of the groove. The edges of the lathe cut donor corner are then tucked into the groove and sutured to hold the tissue lens in place until it is healed onto the cornea. The patient's epithelium grows over the added tissue which is now the new surface of the cornea, making it a permanent contact lens. New biological adhesives have allowed the surgeon to glue the new tissue to the cornea and omit the sutures.

In myopia that is so great that contact lenses will not work, the lenses in spectacles will make things appear much smaller.

Everything is reduced so much that the 20/40 line letters become smaller than the normal 20/20 letters. This is like looking through the wrong end of binoculars. People with very high myopia may only be able to read the 20/50 or 20/60 line on the chart with glasses and they cannot wear contact lenses. It is impossible for them to be able to pass their drivers license vision examination.

Some epikeratophakia patients are able to pass their drivers license exams, for the first time, after this procedure.

The epikeratophakia lens for myopia is thin in the center so it clears rapidly after surgery. A similar procedure was designed for people who had undergone cataract surgery but did not get a replacement intraocular lens. The epikeratophakia lens for correction of the high degree of hyperopia following cataract surgery was thick in the middle and thin in the periphery The drawback to the epikeratophakia correction after cataract surgery was that it took forever to heal and to become optically clear enough to see through.

Sometimes it took a year. Patients were very impatient with the slow healing. We needed a faster result in today's world.

Intracorneal implants]

Since bulging the peripheral cornea causes the central cornea to flatten, a technique was developed to insert curved plastic rods in the peripheral cornea to push the surface forward. Two curved rods formed a ring in the cornea which changed the optical power to treat myopia. This procedure is popular in parts of the country, but is not widely used.

Intraocular lenses

The modern way to correct vision after cataract surgery is to use a small plastic lens which is placed inside the eye during the operation for removal of a cataract. There is a variation in the optical power of the human lens from one patient to the next.

When we implant a lens during cataract removal, we must calculate the correct power of the replacement lens to make the eye focus properly after the surgery. Implant lenses are made in many different powers, usually in 0.50 Diopter steps from +10.00 to +26.00 Diopters. Special lenses are made outside of this range.

Determining the correct power is a mathematics and physics problem using optical principles. Ultrasound and optical measurements of the eye are fed to computer programs that do the calculations in milliseconds. The results are printed out, so the doctor can select the correct lens to make the patient see clearly at a given desired distance without glasses. If the patient was near or farsighted before surgery, we can correct that by choosing the correct lens.

Intraocular lenses are very successful in treating cataracts.

They are high power, plus (+) lenses, put behind the pupil within the remnants of the lens capsule. This is the optimal position for the replacement lens, because it does not magnify or minify what is seen.

Earlier lenses were put in the anterior chamber, in front of the iris. They had feet that were placed in the angle between the cornea and the iris. The optical magnification did not change much from being behind the iris. The length of these lenses had to fit precisely in the eye. If they were short, the lens would move around in the eye creating inflammation which was bad for the eye. Long lenses caused tenderness and pain from the pressure against the angle structures.

Dr. Worst, in Holland, designed a lens with platinum loops, which were pliable and chemically inert. The lens looked like a small contact lens with two loops of wire inserted in the back side. These two loops extended through the pupil and bent at right angles to rest on the back of the iris. As long as the pupil was small, it held the lens centered over the pupil.

Other designs added loops that were in the edge of the lens and extended in front of the iris to keep it from falling backwards into the eye. Many variations were designed including three loops, parallel front and back loops and perpendicular front and back loops, straight wires, called pintles, radiating from the edge of the lens, and prolene (plastic) loops with various shapes.

Ideally, the weight of the lens is exactly offset by the buoyancy of the lens in the fluid of the eye. Platinum loops are heavy so the weight of the lens made it rest on the lower margin of the pupil.

The lens would occasionally fall forward if the pupil dilated.

Plastic loops of Supramid or Prolene were lighter, allowing the buoyancy to balance the weight, making the lens weightless in the eye and better able to stay in place.

Modern lenses are usually placed in the capsule bag at the time of cataract surgery. Dislocation is rare from this location.

Foldable lenses make it possible to insert the five mm. lens through a three mm. cataract surgery incision.

Companies started making minus powered intraocular lenses to place in the anterior chamber to correct high amounts of myopia.

The feet of the lens, being in the angle structures, caused problems so a new lens was developed that clipped onto the iris and did not have feet. This lens is called the claw lens because of the way it grabs the iris.

If the calculation for the lens power that is needed to correct high myopia by removing the human lens yields a power near zero, we can remove the natural lens from the eye and not replace it, allowing distance vision without glasses. In this case, the nearsightedness before surgery is the same amount as the farsightedness produced by removing the human lens so they cancel out.

Small variations from the need for a zero power lens can be easily fixed with conventional glasses after the human lens is removed.

CATARACT

A cataract is defined as opacity of, or within, the human lens. This may be a small speck in the lens, a layer of opacity in the lens, or the entire lens may be cloudy or opaque or yellow-brown in color. (A long standing cataract my even become black.) There are a number of causes for cataracts, including trauma to the eye, electric shock, medications, chemical burns, maternal infection or illness, and systemic disease (diseases that affect the whole body), such as allergies, diabetes, or myotonic dystrophy. The number one cause of cataract is advancing age.

A healthy baby has a very clear and soft lens, like Jell-O, which will continue to grow very slowly throughout life. By the time that child graduates from high school, the clarity of the lens has become mildly translucent, like fish flesh, but light still passes through the lens easily without distortion. By the time that child has reach the age of forty-five, the lens is still translucent, but it has become firm. This firmness prevents it from changing shape to focus the eye, so reading glasses are needed.

As the person approaches sixty or seventy, the protein in the lens begins to turn amber or brown and the outer parts become white. The center of the lens may also become foggy white. Along with this change in color, the protein in the lens changes in optical properties. It bends the light that is passing through it more, making the person more myopic or less hyperopic. The person may now be able to read without reading glasses, but distance vision is blurred. Correcting this myopia with glasses or contact lenses will often restore useful vision and delay the need for cataract surgery. Ethical ophthalmologists will always try to improve vision by correcting the glasses before suggesting cataract surgery.

Eventually, the opacity of the lens becomes so dense that the light is blocked and distorted, so that vision cannot be improved by changing glasses. When the entire lens has turned white or brown, it is considered to be, "mature." If a mature cataract is not removed, the outer layers of the cataract, called the cortex, will eventually dissolve and look like skim milk. This material is held in the lens by the lens capsule, a clear membrane like plastic wrap that holds the lens together. The center part of the cataract, called the nucleus, remains hard and dark brown or black and may settle to the bottom of the capsule bag after the cortex has become liquid.

This is called a hyper mature cataract. Besides possibly causing inflammatory reactions and glaucoma, a hypermature cataract is much more difficult to remove without complications. A mature lens, or the beginning of a hypermature lens, is a cause to remove the cataract. If left in the eye, the liquid cortex may leak from the lens and cause inflammation leading to glaucoma. This leakage may cause either toxic reaction or an immune response.

Another common form of cataract is called the posterior sub capsular cataract. It usually forms in people from age 45 and up, but may occur at younger ages. This type of cataract can be caused by repeated trauma like prize fighting or bar brawling. It starts as fine spots of white, or pearly-white, material in the center of the back surface of the lens. Histologically, these spots are just beneath the back surface of the capsule and usually are aligned with the center of the pupil opening when viewed from the front of the eye. These spots gather and spread out from the center of the back surface. When there are only a few, the eye can see around and between them.

When the eye looks at distance, the pupil enlarges, making it easier to see around the cataract. When the eye looks at near, as when reading, the pupil becomes small and the cataract blocks and scatters more of the light. Many people do not notice the cataract until the day the spot on the back surface of the lens is big enough to block the pupil completely. It seems to have a very sudden onset although it may have been accumulating for many months.

How do I know if I have a cataract? The early symptoms of cataract are: blurred vision, difficulty seeing at night due to glare or flares around lights, (light scattering by the opacities), difficulty reading, (posterior sub capsular cataract blocking the pupil), difficulty with distance vision, (cataract induced myopia), and changes in color vision, (light absorption of certain colors by the darkened lens proteins).

Light shining into the eye from lamps, candles or sunlight will light up the opacities producing glare and making it hard to see through the illuminated haze. This is like high beam headlights in fog or looking through a dirty windshield when the sun shines on it. I have had patients tell me that they cleaned the windshield of their car many times until they realized that the problem was in their eye and not the windshield.

Since cataracts may cause increased myopia without dimming the vision, the ability to see fine print at a closer distance than usual should prompt an examination for cataracts.

The gradual visual loss from a normal age-related cataract may be so slow that it is not noticed until you have an eye examination.

> One lady had lost vision to 20/200 in both eyes and told me that her vision had not changed. She told me that her vision did not affect how she drove her car. I told her that it was not legal for her to drive her car with the vision she had and wrote in the record that she had been told not to drive. A week later she ran over a man at a bank drive up window, killing him. She told the police that she did not see him.
>
> I was glad that I had written in her chart that I had told her not to drive when the dead man's lawyer came

to my office to see why she was still driving after I had examined her. In Texas the doctor can be held liable for an accident if he has not told the patient not to drive when they do not meet the vision criteria for a driver's license.

When should you have a cataract removed? The answer to this question depends on many things. The first is how well you function with your present vision. This assumes that your ophthalmologist has corrected any cataract induced myopia or error in your present glasses.

How well you function depends of your present visual demands. If you do not drive a car or fly an airplane, do not like to read for pleasure, do not have a job that requires accuracy in reading numbers, or you spend most of your time watching television, the removal of the cataract is not urgent. If the cataract is only in one eye and the other eye is good, it depends how much the cataract eye bothers you. If the cataract is in your dominant eye it will probably bother you a lot. If it is in your non-dominant eye, you can probably ignore it until it becomes bad enough to bother you or until the other eye starts getting a cataract.

If you need to drive, like to read a lot, or have a job, such as accounting or publishing, which requires good vision, you may want to have the cataract removed when your vision decreases to 20/40 or below. Twenty/forty is the cut off vision for driving in most states. Some insurance will not pay for the surgery, as being medically necessary, unless your vision is 20/40 or worse.

In a darkened ophthalmology office it is easier to read the eye chart than in a brightly lighted room which is more like your daily living environment or office. Some ophthalmologists actually shine a light in your eye and ask you to read the chart to see the effect of glare on your vision; so-called glare testing. Glare is a big problem with night driving. Oncoming headlights light up the cataract, making it difficult to see through. If you have to drive at night, you may need to have your cataract removed earlier than if you do not drive at night.

Another consideration in older people is being able to see well enough to avoid falls. A cataract in one eye may interfere with three dimensional vision and depth perception. Not being able to see the height of a curb or step can cause a fall with a possible hip or pelvic fracture. Not being able to judge distances while cooking may lead to burns from mistakes in pouring or touching hot objects.

You must decide how much you are impaired by your decreased vision. If it interferes with your lifestyle, you should strongly consider having the cataract removed. Inactivity from poor vision may lead to general physical and psychological decline.

Driven partly by efficiency and partly by greed, some ophthalmologists are urging their patients to have both cataracts removed one week apart. Some doctors fear that if the first eye does not come out to your expectations that you will go to another doctor for the second eye. One week after surgery is too soon for you to tell how the first operation will come out.

It is now generally accepted that having both cataracts removed at the same operation is an invitation to disaster. If this happens, and things do not go well, the doctor will almost always lose in court. If there is contamination in the operating theater or the autoclave is not working properly, you could get an infection in both eyes and loose them both. If you fall during the first few weeks after the surgery and rupture the wound, it could lead to the loss of the eye. If both eyes have fresh incisions, both could be lost. People often have poor vision for a few weeks after surgery that could cause a loss of depth perception and subsequently lead to a fall. If both eyes have been operated and have temporary poor vision, the chances of falls increase.

The operated eye may not see well for several weeks after surgery. Glasses are not usually fit until three to six weeks after surgery to allow the incision to heal and the optics of the eye to stabilize. During that time you may have to depend of the non operated eye. By six weeks, your vision with the operated eye may be so good that you can put off surgery on the other eye until the poor vision from it interferes with your good eye, especially if the surgery was in your dominant eye. Many inactive older people may do just fine after having one cataract removed and never need to have the second cataract surgery. Active people will usually want both eyes corrected to have better depth perception and a wider field of vision.

How long should I wait to do the second cataract? I recommend at least six weeks to three months. Most complications of cataract surgery occur within the first few weeks after surgery.

One reason for this delay for the second eye is a complication that occurs, not infrequently, that is hard to predict. This complication, called cystoid macular edema or CME, happens at about six weeks to three months after successful cataract surgery. It is more common after complications like capsule tears and vitreous loss.

The vision rapidly becomes blurred and color vision may be lost in the operated eye. This is caused by a swelling in the retina, especially the macula. This swelling may persist for several weeks, or rarely, up to a year, before it spontaneously clears and vision returns. CME is most common in blond, blue eyed, patients of northern European descent (Scandinavian, Germanic, etc.).

People who have this problem in the first operated eye have it more often than average in the second eye when it is operated. If both eyes are operated within the three month period and both develop CME, the person could have very poor vision in both eyes for up to a year. This vision is often much worse during CME than the vision in the unoperated eye, so the person is much worse off than if they had delayed the surgery on the second eye.

The use of non-steroidal anti-inflammatory drugs, NSAIDs, before and after surgery, has reduced the frequency of this complication, but not prevented it completely. In my experience, most treatment is ineffective once the edema has occurred.

If the first eye has not developed this retinal edema by three months after the surgery and the operated eye sees well, it is very unlikely that the CME will occur in the operated eye, so surgery can proceed in the second eye.

What is cataract surgery like? Modern day cataract surgery is much better and faster that when our parents had it done. When my grandfather had cataract surgery, the cataract had to be "ripe" or "mature." That meant that the whole lens had to have become white or brownish white. Vision in that eye was "bumping into the wall" vision.

This extreme criteria was because the techniques used at that time required the patient to lie in bed for three weeks with heavy sandbags taped to his/her head to keep them from moving until the wound was healed enough not to rupture when the patient exerted to get out of bed.

Being confined to bed for three weeks can cause an old person to lose calcium from their bones, which leads to osteoporosis and fractures. Under these conditions a person may break a hip by merely standing up and putting weight on their legs.

Lying on your back for three weeks will cause pooling of fluid in the back and bases of the lungs. This fluid is a rich bed for infection to develop and may lead to pneumonia that can be fatal.

Another complication of lying in bed for three weeks is the formation of blood clots in the legs. These clots can break loose and move to the heart and lungs creating a fatal pulmonary embolism. People used to die from complications of cataract extraction.

> Shortly after I arrived in Texas, a post cataract surgery patient was brought to the clinic after five days in the hospital after cataract surgery. He was transported to the clinic by wheel chair and walked a few steps to the examination chair. Shortly after he sat in the chair, he slumped forward and passed out. He had no heart beat so we started CPR.

Our attempts to start his heart were unsuccessful and he died. The postmortem examination showed that CPR would not have worked, because he had a large pulmonary embolism that obstructed the pulmonary artery that went from his heart to the lungs. It had broken loose from his calf when he walked from the wheel chair to the exam chair. It had rapidly passed from his leg through his heart and on to plug the pulmonary artery.

Present day cataract surgery takes about half an hour and is done as an outpatient. The old complications from bed rest have essentially disappeared. Modern surgical techniques are different; the suture material is much better; the surgery is more carefully done under the surgical microscope, and incisions are smaller, resulting in better wound closure and fewer complications.

What preparation is necessary for cataract surgery? If you decide to have cataract surgery, the eye to be operated must be measured to determine the power of the implant lens to be used.

Ultrasound is used to measure the optical length of the eyeball and the position of the new lens. The curvature and optical power of the cornea is determined using a keratometer. These numbers are entered into a computer that prints out a list of lens powers and the resulting optical correction needed for that lens. The doctor then decides which power will work best and orders that lens for the surgery. Usually, several lenses are chosen to deal with various complications that may arise during surgery. A lens placed in front of the iris, the fallback position, will require a different power than one placed in the usual place, the capsule bag.

The doctor may order antibiotic eye drops for you to put in the eye for one to three days before the surgery. The night before surgery you may be asked to wash your face with surgical soap.

We used to cut off the eyelashes on the eye to be operated. This reduced the numbers of bacteria around the eye and marked the eye to be operated. The plastic drapes that are now used around the eye to prepare the surgical field cover the lashes, so most doctors no longer cut the lashes before surgery. Lashes take three to six weeks to grow back after surgery. Since the recuperation period is so short now, most surgeons and patients do not want any signs of the surgery after the first few days and do not want their lashes clipped.

Depending on your health and the requirements of the outpatient surgery unit, you may have to have blood work, a urinalysis, an electrocardiogram, a chest X-ray, and an examination by your general physician to assure the surgeon and the anesthesiologist that you are well enough to have surgery.

On the morning of surgery you are not to eat or drink anything.

If you take medications, your doctor may allow you to take them with sips of water—just enough to be able to swallow them.

If you are a diabetic on insulin, your doctor or the anesthesiologist will tell you how much insulin to take on the morning of surgery, possibly none. If you take medications during the day, you should bring them with you in case the surgery, or your discharge from the surgery unit, is delayed.

What happens during cataract surgery? On the day of surgery, you report to the outpatient surgery unit. Great pains are taken to identify you and determine which eye is to be operated. The eye is marked with an indelible pen so the mark is not washed off during the preparation of the operated area. The nurses will start an intravenous infusion and several eye drops will be instilled into the eye to be operated. These drops are used to dilate the pupil and sterilize the surface of the eye and eye lids.

Some surgeons give an injection around and behind the eye to numb the eye and keep it from moving during the surgery.

They may wait until you are in the surgery room before giving the nerve block. Some doctors use only topical anesthesia, so there is no shot. Topical anesthesia is less reliable, but it is popular because there is no painful injection.

I preferred to make an injection to the eyelids to keep the patient from blinking or squeezing the eyelids during surgery. I gave an injection behind the eye to paralyze the ocular muscles so the eye could not move during surgery and the eye would not feel any pain from the surgery. Since the incision is only two or three millimeters long and is usually plugged by an instrument, many surgeons have abandoned these two injections. They prefer to use numbing eye drops and to irrigate an anesthetic into the eye to numb it for surgery.

Once in the operating room, the nurses will check again to see which eye is to be operated. Many operating rooms will "call a time out." All activity in the operating room stops until everyone present agrees on which eye is to be operated. The area around the eye will be washed with antiseptic solution and then drapes will be applied to cover all of you, head to toe, except the eye to be operated. The nurse or the surgeon will move the microscope into position and adjust the focus and magnification.

A speculum will be placed in the eye to hold the eyelids open and to expose the eye for surgery. The eye is usually irrigated with saline solution to remove any prep solution, mucus or loose eyelashes.

Some surgeons use a silver protein solution, Argyrol, to sterilize the surface of the eyeball and coagulate any mucus that coats the eye. This coagulum is wiped from the eye.

Because of the intravenous sedation, you may be asleep by now and not be aware of what is happening until they wake you up at the end of the surgery. Some people are hyper enough that they do not sleep, but are mildly content from the anesthesia.

The sedation usually makes you amnesic for everything that happened since the sedation was started until it wears off.

> I had one patient who was extremely nervous. She was sedated for her first cataract surgery which went well.

When I operated on the second eye, one year later, she kept telling me that I was doing things differently than for her first eye. She did not remember my giving her an injection or putting on the drapes. My routine had not varied, but the sedation during her first operation had made her forget what I had done.

At this point of the surgery, techniques vary. Different incisions and different techniques are used to remove the cataract.

Sometimes sutures are necessary, but usually the wound is so small and constructed in such a way that it can be left to be self sealing, called "no stitch" surgery. Some surgeons use "one stitch" surgery. That means that only one suture stitch is used, but that one stitch may be a figure eight or shoelace pattern with multiple closure points. The old techniques required seven or more stitches to close a longer incision.

Most ophthalmologists now use phacoemulsification to remove the cataract. This technique uses a sharp hypodermic needle, bent at the tip, to tear a smooth edged, round hole in the front surface of the lens capsule to expose the body of the lens.

(Now an expensive laser can be used to make this opening.) Fluid is injected into the lens to separate the hard center or nucleus from the soft cortex, freeing the nucleus. The nucleus can be left in the lens capsule, or delivered into the front of the eye to be broken into small pieces. A hollow needle that vibrates at five thousand vibrations a second, ultrasound frequency, is used to sculpt away the exposed lens core. The needle is used in various patterns, depending on the preference of the surgeon to break the lens into tiny pieces that can be sucked from the eye through the hollow vibrating needle.

Fluid is constantly irrigated into the eye to replace the fluid being removed with the lens particles. After the core of the lens is removed, a different needle is used to peel away the outer layers of the cataract that still adhere to the inside of the capsule. As much as possible of the lens cortex is removed, leaving the empty capsule bag. It is like a trampoline, suspended from the ciliary body behind the pupil by about one hundred tiny threads called suspensory ligaments, or zonules. There are various techniques used to insert a small plastic lens into the capsule bag to replace the optical power of the lens (cataract) that was removed. The capsule bag holds the new lens behind the iris, centered in the pupil. If the capsule ruptures during the operation, the replacement lens may be placed in front of the iris, resting on the angle structures, or it can be sutured in place behind the iris.

Some doctors give injections of antibiotics and/or steroids around the eye at the end of the surgery. Some patch the operated eye; others insert a soft bandage lens to protect the eye until the anesthetic wears off.

Most ocular surgeons insist on seeing the patient the next day in their office. However, it is becoming more common that the patient is seen by a technician or physician's assistant rather than the surgeon. This visit is to check the wound for proper closure, check the pressure in the eye and look for signs of infection.

A viscous material called viscoelastic is used during surgery to fill the front of the eye to hold the iris and lens back from the cornea, to provide working space for the instruments, and to protect the cornea. The first material that was used was made from rooster combs and was called Healon. Healon has become the "generic" name used by most doctors for this and similar materials (the same way we use Kleenex for tissue and Frigidaire for refrigerator). It is irrigated from the eye at the end of surgery, but some of it may remain in the eye. The thick viscosity of this material may cause it to temporarily block the outflow channels, raising the intraocular pressure for one to three days. If the pressure is too high, the doctor will prescribe eye drops to lower it.

When I trained in the seventies, we kept the patient in the hospital for five days and saw them every day, once or twice each day. Our biggest problem was poor wound closure with leaks of aqueous humor from the eye resulting in low intraocular pressure.

We also looked closely for early signs of infection in the eye.

Better wound closure and better antibiotics have decreased the need for daily visits after surgery.

It is important that the patient monitors the way the eye feels and contacts the doctor if there is pain or rough feeling in the eye. Once vision is good enough to see images, the patient should watch for changes in vision, other than improvement. The presence of flashes or shadows might indicate a retinal detachment.

Pain or blurring of vision may indicate infection within the eye.

Although rare, retinal detachment is one of the most common complications of cataract surgery. It causes the appearance of shadows or curtains in the visual area.

Some doctors restrict activities for several days or up to three weeks after surgery. The patient should not bend forward at the waist, lift anything over 20 pounds, or get on their hands and knees (washing floors or hunting lost objects). Many physicians do not want the patient to drive for several weeks following surgery.

This is partially because of decreased vision in the operated eye and loss of depth perception to judge distances and partially because a sudden movement like slamming on the brakes or swerving to avoid a collision might strain or bump the eye and reposition the wound edges or implant lens.

Some surgeons place no restrictions at all on their patients, because the new procedures use small incisions or the incision is sutured with strong suture material. I believe in some mild restrictions because I was trained when the restrictions were significant and had good reasons behind them. Many of those reasons still apply today.

> I removed a cataract on a ninety-two-year-old lawyer who still walked several blocks to the office each day, mostly to check the mail and talk with his partners. The day after surgery he asked me how soon he could resume his daily activity of ten push-ups every morning when he

got out of bed. I hated to tell him not to do it for at least three weeks, because I was surprised that a man of his age could still do ten push-ups every morning. His push-ups would raise intraocular pressure and put him in a face down position.

Both should be avoided for several weeks after cataract surgery. I told him to wait three weeks.

One new precaution that arose with the use of implant lenses is the caveat not to read for forty-eight hours after the surgery.

The intraocular lens that is used to replace the optical power of the cataract is usually placed in the bag of the capsule that is left after the opaque part of the lens is removed. After several days, the front and back parts of the capsule will collapse together and fuse around the lens positioning loops, holding the lens in place.

During the first two or three days, some of the viscoelastic material may be left in the capsule bag, holding it open and allowing the lens to move. The viscoelastic will dissolve in two or three days, allowing the front and back parts of the capsule to come in contact to hold the lens.

Reading involves slow movements of the eyes from word to word toward the right followed by fast movement to the left to start the next line. The slow, short, movements will not move the lens, but the fast return movement may cause the lens to shift within the capsule. This movement, repeated many times in reading a newspaper or a book may cause the lens to move off center.

Studies of people watching television have shown that the eyes move around the screen randomly and do not have a repeating pattern that might displace a lens. Watching TV is permitted.

The surgical wound must knit together and heal. If there are sutures, they will slowly relax as the wound heals and as the sutures slowly cut through the tissue, because they are tight. This process takes three to six weeks. The changes in wound healing and suture relaxation cause the shape of the cornea to change.

An incision that has not been sutured, as in "no stitch" surgery, will relax and then contract over the same period of time. This movement may cause improvement or deterioration in the vision without glasses, and it eventually influences the strength of the corrective spectacle lenses that may be needed after surgery.

The cataractous lens often filters different colors of light to varying degrees. People with cataracts will comment that they cannot see red traffic lights very well. Spouses comment that their husband or wife cannot pick out their clothes very well and often get color mismatches. After cataract removal, people remark that colors are much brighter, especially the blue shades.

Colors through the cataract are brownish and muddy. Some people want the second eye done immediately so that the colors from the two eyes do not clash.

> A patient of mine who had a blue tourmaline stone in her ring told me that she thought she had been swindled because the color of her ring never changed. Tourmaline is supposed to change color, between blue and purple, when going from sunlight to artificial light. She told me after having her cataract removed that the color change was very vivid from blue to purple.

The human lens filters ultraviolet light from the light entering the eye. Ultraviolet light is harmful to the retina. The intraocular lenses used after cataract extraction contain chemicals that filter and block ultraviolet light so the retina is not damaged by sunlight after a cataract has been removed.

The human lens also removes infrared light, including heat waves. People who work near high temperatures, like glass blowers and welders, may develop cataracts from the infrared light.

When the human lens is removed from the eye, the person can see better in the dark. This was a military secret during World War I. The Allies used old people, who had had their cataracts removed, as night spotters for snipers. They could see the body heat of soldiers hiding in trees, bushes, or windows of buildings at night and point them out to the snipers. The body heat was infrared radiation (light).

At about six weeks after surgery the doctor will determine if glasses are needed, and if so, what strength. If there was significant astigmatism before surgery, glasses may be needed to correct that after surgery. Because the eye was cut and manipulated during surgery, the lens that was carefully calculated before surgery may not give the perfect result after everything heals. The computer calculation is reported to one one-hundredth of a Diopter, the lenses only come in fifty, one hundredth steps (0.50 Diopters).

The measurements of the eye that the doctor, or technician, does are difficult to make with complete accuracy. If they are incorrect by a small amount, it may throw off the power of the lens by enough to make a difference in the vision after surgery.

This inaccuracy can be easily corrected with spectacles. For some people, the slight decrease from perfect vision without glasses may be tolerated. If the implant lens is significantly different than what is needed, a lens exchange for a better lens can be performed surgically.

Intraocular lenses, IOL, implant

Before implant lenses, people who had cataracts removed usually wore thick cataract glasses that magnified everything they saw by about thirty percent. By moving the focusing power of the human lens from behind the pupil to a spectacle lens in front of the eye, the optical physics of the new position cause the image to be magnified. The power of a lens needed to focus light on the back of the eye changes as the lens is moved farther away from the eye. Higher power lenses magnify more.

Before intraocular lenses, if someone had one cataract removed they could not use both eyes together with glasses after surgery.

The image from the unoperated eye is normal in size while the operated eye sees a magnified image. The brain could not put the two images from the different eyes together to make one picture.

They would see double images—one large, one regular sized.

When you looked at steps, you would see a large set of steps and a normal sized set of steps. Which one do you put your foot on?

(Actually, when they look at their feet, they have two sets, one normal and one large. Simply put one large foot on the large step and one small foot will automatically be on the small step. This is still disconcerting.)

This problem caused many falls. People had to choose which eye they wanted to use. Most people chose the eye that had not been operated unless the corrected vision in the operated eye was much better than the corrected vision in the normal eye. Studies showed that using the familiar sized vision was preferred until the operated eye saw better than the not operated eye by five lines on the eye chart.

Part of the dissatisfaction with the operated eye was that the glasses were only good for the central thirty to forty degrees of vision. Since the cataract glasses magnified by thirty percent, turning your head caused one hundred and thirty percent of the world to pass by. The world seemed to move in the opposite direction. This made people dizzy, another cause for falls.

The cataract glasses magnified everything that was seen through them by about thirty percent. This made the image larger than life so it overlapped what was seen around the lens. It was possible for someone to approach the person wearing cataract glasses, within the blind spot between the magnified image and the blurred surrounding area. They could approach the person until they were too large to fit in the blind spot and then they popped out, several feet in front of the person. This was frightening to the person. It was called the "Jack-in-the-box" phenomenon.

One of my professors said that older people tend to be paranoid about people surprising them and this appearance of people very close to them made it worse.

Some people wore contact lenses because contacts only magnified about five percent. The brain could fuse that slightly enlarged picture with the regular sized picture from the normal eye. Many older people, the age when cataracts occur, could not handle contacts because of arthritis or nervousness. Some thought contacts were just for young people who were vain, so they refused to try them.

Intraocular lenses for cataract surgery were a godsend. Since they are placed at, or near, the same position where the original lens had been, there is no optical magnification or distortion.

The operated eye works well with the one that was not operated.

By eliminating the problem of different image sizes in the two eyes we can delay cataract operation on the second eye until the vision in that eye has deteriorated. Before that, people who had a cataract removed were disappointed when they did not use the operated eye after surgery, but continued to rely on the other eye.

Intraocular lenses do not restore the eye to the youthful state.

These plastic lenses do not focus in and out. If the lenses are calculated for distance, which is customary, reading glasses are needed for reading and near work. There are new intraocular lenses that have been designed to focus in and out to remove the need for reading glasses, or any glasses at all. These lenses depend on flexing of the lens to move it forward and backward in the eye to focus for distance and near, or they are designed as multifocal lenses with part of the lens focused at distance and part focused at near. These new lenses are approved by the FDA, but I feel that they are still somewhat experimental. Not everyone with one of these lenses can throw away their glasses.

I worry that in patients with both eyes operated with these new lenses that the two eyes may not be focused together at distance or near and that the images will fight in the brain for dominance and may cause headaches.

The Z syndrome has been reported. The intraocular lens is supposed to fold from front to back, both above and below, so the lens moves forward and backward as the ciliary body contracts and expands. This forward and backward movement focuses the eye in and out. In the Z syndrome, one end of the folding lens bends the wrong way forming a Z shape, rather than the shape of a capital C. Contraction or expansion of the ciliary body ring pushes one end forward and the other backward resulting in a the tilt of the lens, but it does not move the optical part forward or backward in the eye. This changes the astigmatism in the eye, but not the focus. There are various surgical procedures to correct this error in lens folding, if it occurs.

How do I choose a cataract surgeon? Medicine has become a competitive business, rather than a noble profession. The old social contract of professionals, like doctors and lawyers, was that the ethics of the professions protected citizens from being taken advantage of by the professionals, so the citizens held the professions in high regard. In the current age, doctors advertize to get more patients. Some, unethically, claim to be the best surgeons or use better equipment or techniques than other doctors. The best technique should be the one which produces the best result for the patient in the hands of a particular surgeon. The goal should be to get the best results for the patient, not the most profit for the practice or the most prestige, because of the popularity of a new technique. Whether the surgeon uses a knife or a laser for the incision or uses sutures to close the incision, or not, should not be a deciding factor in selecting an ophthalmic surgeon.

Just because a TV ad says that a doctor is the best, does not mean that they are. A doctor, who has to advertise for patients, may need to advertize because they do not have a good reputation among the doctors who refer patients. Some have big egos and feel that they are saving the patients from going to other surgeons, who they do not think are as good as they are.

I feel that a good doctor is humble enough to realize that there are other doctors as good or better than they are, but is self confident enough to know that they can give the best care to their patients.

If you have been going to an ophthalmologist that you like who does cataract surgery, you should probably stay with them.

Talk to patients in the waiting room when you go to see him/her to see if they are satisfied with the results and the way they were treated.

If you hear bad things about a doctor, consider the source. If the stories are consistently bad, find another doctor you can trust.

Doctor/patient trust is important in the medical situation. It is perfectly alright to ask a surgeon if they have done the procedure before and approximately how many they have done. If your doctor does not have time to talk to you about the surgery he is recommending, he may not be around if you have complications.

Most of the grading systems for physicians that are available today do not accurately evaluate the physicians they grade. They use patient volume, office appearance, and waiting time and billing complaints to base their evaluations, not surgical results, personality, and ability to cope with complications. These are the things that really matter.

Ask friends and family for recommendations for doctors with whom they have had experience. Whether the doctor is in a group or in solo practice does not make a difference. Every ophthalmologist who has trained in the past thirty years has been taught how to remove cataracts in the modern way. People trained before then and still in practice have a lot of experience.

Every doctor, no matter how good or well trained, can have complications during and after surgery. No two people are exactly the same and results may vary, so outcomes are not guaranteed.

Cataract surgery is one of the most successful operations in all of medicine, but not everyone gets a perfect result. People are all different in many small ways. Despite what the medical managers tell us, one size fits all medicine does not work. Sometimes it is necessary to go to plan "B" or plan "C" before good results are obtained. Not everyone responds the same way to a particular treatment.

It amazed me, when phacoemulsification was first introduced, that doctors were going to weekend courses, practicing on two or three rabbit eyes, and returning home with their new, forty thousand dollar phacoemulsification machine to do surgery on their patients. Many eyes were blinded by these surgeons who thought they could learn a very complex surgical procedure in a weekend and do it without practice.

When phacoemulsification first was being taught, I was at the University of Texas in Galveston. Dr. Ferguson and I had gone to a "phaco" course and then practiced on a number of rabbits and cats to perfect our technique. The course provided two rabbit eyes and one cat eye for each doctor enrolled in the course.

Most of the participants did one or two practice eyes and left. Dr. Ferguson and I used all of the unused eyes so we each did about eight practice eyes. When we returned to Galveston, we each did several more practice eyes.

The university wanted to have a "university without walls," offering courses to graduates to teach new techniques and new medical techniques. We had an animal surgery laboratory which was used for research. It had all of the equipment needed to practice new surgical procedures, including video taping of microscopic surgery for self critique. We had a popular type of "phaco" machine. We advertized a one to three day intensive practice session with tutoring and video feedback at a moderate cost. No one signed up for the course.

I continued to see patients who needed corneal transplants or vitrectomy to treat the complications of inexperienced "Phaco" surgeons. I did vitrectomies to remove lens fragments from the back of the eye and clean up the mess left behind by these inexperienced surgeons. I learned of surgeons who were so frustrated that they pushed the new machine into the corner of the operating room and abandoned the procedure, going back to the prior methods of removing cataracts. This disappointed the hospital administrators who had purchased these very expensive machines that were not being used.

Ophthalmologists practicing today have either been trained during residency to do phacoemulsification or have had years to adopt this procedure, so there is no worry about untrained eye surgeons now.

Complications of cataract surgery

The complications of cataract surgery used to be pneumonia, pulmonary emboli, broken hips, wound rupture, leaking eyes, retinal detachment, and blindness. With the advances in technique, better suture materials, microsurgery, improved medications, and outpatient surgery, the type and incidence of complications have changed.

Outpatient surgery has all but eliminated the problems of pneumonia, emboli and broken hips. Better wound closure (because of use of the microscope), different incisions, (because of different cataract removal techniques), and better suture materials have eliminated wound leaks and wound rupture and also reduced the incidence of retinal detachment.

New complications have arisen, like elevated intraocular pressure from tighter wound closure and the use of viscous, space holding, materials (Healon) that block the outflow channels.

Cystoid macular edema (CME) that follows cataract surgery by several months was described by Irvine and Gass in 1953 and has slowly become more prevalent. The increase in incidence of CME has been correlated to the increase in the incidence of women wearing Nylon stockings. This means that we do not really know what causes CME. It now occurs in up to thirty percent of post operative cataracts, especially in patients with diabetes or other retinal vascular problems. Complications such as vitreous loss and capsule rupture have been shown to increase the probability of getting CME. The use of NSAIDs and smaller incisions may have decreased the incidence of CME.

The combination of intraocular lenses and phacoemulsification has brought a new set of complications. Intraocular lenses can be dislocated within the eye and cause problems with glaucoma, and inflammation. Phacoemulsification has increased the number of corneas that fail after cataract extraction. Corneal transplants are used to replace the damaged corneas. The technique of phacoemulsification has led to more ruptured lens capsules with loss of some of the lens into the back of the eye. Lens fragments in the vitreous gel must be removed before they cause inflammation and damage to the eye. The incidence of retinal detachment is much higher in patients with torn capsules and displaced lens fragments or leaking wounds.

Hemorrhage

Hemorrhage into the front of the eye is usually a minor complication after cataract surgery. If a vessel is cut in the process of making the incision, it will usually spasm and shut off the flow of blood. After the surgery, the muscle spasm may relax and allow blood to flow from the severed blood vessel into the eye until a clot forms to stop the bleeding. The collection of blood in the front of the eye is called a post operative hyphema. It will usually flow out of the eye through the outflow channels during the next three to five days, leaving no residual problem.

> I had a patient with a cataract who was from out of town.
>
> He came to me during the early use of intraocular lenses.
>
> He was very active and played handball every week. He did not like contact lenses and had only one cataract so cataract glasses would not work. He had heard of intraocular lenses and wanted one to replace his cataract.

This was before the modern posterior chamber lenses.

We were worried that if we put a pupil supported lens in his eye that it might be displaced by strenuous activity or trauma from playing handball. We decided to place a rigid plastic lens in his anterior chamber between the iris and the cornea. These lenses have rigid feet that extend into the angle structures where the iris and cornea come together, making them very stable.

His surgery went smoothly. The night after surgery the patient was still in the hospital. At about 2:00 AM, he was awakened by pain in his eye. The resident was called immediately to examine the eye and found a significant hemorrhage in the anterior chamber of the eye, surrounding the implant lens. This hemorrhage recurred on the next three nights at about the same time causing the pressure in the eye to go up.

High pressure can drive the red blood cells into the cornea where they break down and stain the cornea with hemoglobin. The hemoglobin will slowly disappear, but it may take up to a year to clear enough to restore vision.

We decided to remove the lens and the blood from the front of the eye before blood staining could occur.

In the operating room, I reopened the incision and slid the implant lens from the eye. A blood clot remained in the eye, so I used the Roto-extractor, an instrument with an irrigation and aspiration needle that nibbled the clot along with any vitreous gel, to remove the clot. We did not replace the lens and the hemorrhage did not recur.

Since the hemorrhage usually occurred at about 2 AM, I concluded that he was having REM sleep (Rapid Eye Movement Sleep). The REM sleep jiggled the eye and caused the lens foot to break a blood vessel. REM sleep occurs during deep sleep and is most common at about 2 AM. Since his hemorrhages occurred at about 2 AM each time, it was probably REM sleep, along with the implant lens, that caused them.

Three weeks after the removal of the implant lens, I used a special lens with mirrors to look at the area where the hemorrhage had occurred. I found a small blood vessel that had grown across the angle where the foot of the lens had been resting in the angle. This was probably the source of the bleeding. Some patients have one or more of these vessels that occur normally.

The patient decided to wear a contact lens to correct his vision after removal of his natural lens. He called me six weeks later to tell me that he was wearing his contact lens and seeing well enough to play handball once a week.

Hemorrhage into the eye can be much worse if it occurs in the back of the eye. Hemorrhage under the retina can cause the contents of the eye to be forced out through an open incision.

This is known as an expulsive hemorrhage.

When the eye is opened, the pressure in the eye becomes the same as the atmosphere, a significant decrease from the closed eye state. We try to minimize this difference by massaging the eye after the block is placed until the eye is soft. If the pressure drops suddenly as the incision is made, the blood pressure in the vessels does not change, so the difference between pressure inside blood vessels and the pressure on the outside of the vessel becomes much greater.

Arteries, or arterioles, that have developed atherosclerosis, hardening of the arteries, may burst because of this sudden loss in the pressure on the outside of the vessel. The arterioles that enter the back of the eye near the optic nerve to supply the choroidal vascular bed are particularly susceptible to atherosclerosis and are the most likely to burst during surgery. This causes hemorrhage to spread behind the retina and choroid pushing everything forward within the eye. If the incision is open, the pressure pushes the lens, iris and vitreous out of the eye. If not detected early and treated appropriately, the eye will be lost.

> The first cataract operation that I performed resulted in an expulsive hemorrhage. A hypermature cataract had caused inflammation and high pressure in the eye. The high pressure and inflammation mandated removal of the cataract. The pressure and inflammation predisposed the eye to an expulsive hemorrhage. Because of the hemorrhage, the vision was lost in that eye. I learned how not to treat expulsive hemorrhage and, during the following several weeks, how to successfully treat it the next time it occurred.

I soon learned that expulsive hemorrhages occur in about 1 in ten thousand cataract operations in non inflamed eyes. I reasoned that I had about nine thousand nine hundred and ninety-nine cataract operations to go before my next expulsive hemorrhage.

Because of the number of complicated cases I operated, including many "lost eyes," my career incidence was greater than one in ten thousand. Fortunately I was able to save most of them.

Infection

One of the most dreaded complications of cataract surgery is infection within the eye. This is called endophthalmitis. We usually have the patient take antibiotic eye drops for several days before surgery to kill any bacteria that are on the outside of the eye or the eyelids. At the time of surgery, a drop of Betadine or Argyrol is placed in the eye to kill any remaining bacteria. This is to prevent live bacteria from being introduced into the eye through the incision.

To create endophthalmitis bacteria must enter the eye. Fluid can be sucked into the eye when the incision is opened. Bacteria may travel into the eye on instruments or in solutions that are injected into the eye in the course of surgery. There have been several epidemics of endophthalmitis from the use of poorly functioning operating room sterilizers when supposedly sterile instruments were contaminated by bacteria and not adequately sterilized.

There was an epidemic of endophthalmitis caused by a batch of contaminated intraocular lenses resulting from an inadequate system of liquid lens sterilization. That system is no longer in use. More commonly, the air conditioning in the operating suite is contaminated and spreads bacteria through the air, causing multiple infections. Hospitals usually test the air in the operating rooms for contamination to avoid this problem. The head of the patient is positioned in the operating room at the "sterile wall." This is the wall farthest from the doors where bacteria might enter.

Infection in the eye causes significant pain in the eye by the second day after surgery. There are signs within the eye such as haziness, floating white blood cells, and dilated blood vessels. To adequately diagnose the type of infection, we must aspirate some fluid from the eye and culture it. We do not wait to find out what the organism is, but inject a combination of antibiotics into the eye at the same time that we aspirate the fluid to culture, usually through the same needle to avoid two needle sticks into the eye.

If we have chosen the correct antibiotics, the patient will notice significant relief of pain within eight hours. We must sometimes repeat the injection of antibiotics at eight to twelve hours after the first injection. We also give the antibiotics by mouth and/or intravenously to treat the retina and anterior eye. The vitreous and the blood eye barrier do not allow the antibiotic to spread from the retina, so injection into the vitreous is the best way to deliver the antibiotics.

When there is not significant pain relief within eight hours, a second injection with antibiotics with a different spectrum of bacterial sensitivity is done at that time.

If the vitreous is very cloudy it usually means that the infection is well established at the time it is seen by the doctor. It may be necessary to remove the vitreous gel, with the organisms within it, to reduce the number of bacteria and to allow better spread of the antibiotics to stop the infection.

The severity of the infection is usually determined by the bacteria that cause it. Some bacteria will cause very little reaction and are sensitive to most antibiotics. Other bacteria are very virulent and can destroy the eye within twenty-four to forty-eight hours. More and more bacteria are becoming resistant to antibiotics, making it harder to cure these infections. Using a dose that is too low to kill the bacteria allows the bacteria to activate enzymes and other mechanisms to make it immune to that particular antibiotic. Overuse of antibiotics allows more exposure to mutations in the bacteria that promote adaptation of the bacteria to the antibiotic.

Corneal Edema

The cornea is the clear window that forms the front of the eye.

The clarity of that window depends on the thin layer of cells that line the back side. This layer, the endothelium, is formed before birth and has the ability to grow and replenish itself for only a short time after birth. After that time, it will no longer be able to repair or replace damaged cells. A child will have about 3500 cells per square millimeter. Slow attrition by trauma and individual cell death decreases that number to about 2500 cells per square millimeter by age sixty. Most corneas with fewer than 2000 cells per square millimeter have corneal edema and loss of clarity. Attempts to establish a minimum number of cells needed to maintain the clarity of the cornea have not been able to come up with that number. Trauma to the eye may also decrease the number of cells on a cornea.

The cells in the endothelial layer are tightly bound together to form a relative barrier to the flow of aqueous humor from the inside of the eye into the cornea. Some fluid is transported from the anterior chamber into the cornea, bringing the metabolic needs of the cornea. This is how the cornea receives nourishment.

There are no blood vessels in a normal cornea.

The endothelial cells also have an active pump mechanism that pumps water out of the cornea, into the eye. When there are too few cells to pump, or there is a breakdown in the barrier, the fluid leaks into the cornea faster than it is removed, causing the cornea to swell and become cloudy, decreasing vision.

Damage to the corneal endothelium from surgery, by touching the endothelium or forceful irrigation, may allow the ocular fluid to leak into the cornea. The cornea absorbs water and will swell and form tiny blisters on the surface of the corneal epithelium, making the surface hazy. This is called corneal edema.

Cataract surgery may damage the corneal endothelium so much that the cornea swells. The tiny micro-blisters make the surface of the cornea like etched glass. The blisters may coalesce to form larger blisters that break when the eyelid blinks. Since the corneal surface has a very high concentration of nerves, this can be very painful, especially when there are many blisters.

Steroid eye drops improve the barrier function of the endothelial layer. The endothelial cells may spread and migrate to cover damaged areas to restore the barrier. If this spreading and migration is not sufficient, the cornea remains swollen and the blisters continue to break. The cornea does not make new endothelial cells after infancy.

A few people undergoing cataract surgery have an underlying disease, Fuch's dystrophy, which causes loss of endothelial cells and separation of the endothelial cells. The leakage between cells and the lack of enough healthy endothelial cells to pump the leaked fluid back out of the cornea can eventually lead to corneal edema. If this disease is not detected before cataract surgery, the trauma of surgery may cause the cornea to decompensate and go into frank corneal edema. The ophthalmologist must look for irregularities in the endothelium called guttata which are the hallmark of Fuch's dystrophy. Extra steps during surgery may avoid later corneal edema.

Another measure of the health of the cornea is the thickness of the cornea. There are optical and electronic means of measuring the thickness. The normal thickness of the center of the human cornea is 0.54 millimeters. If the cornea is more than 0.60 millimeters thick, it is significantly impaired and may decompensate after cataract surgery.

Once the cornea decompensates, it stays cloudy, because it cannot produce new endothelial cells. The only way to make it work again is to replace the corneal endothelium with new tissue.

This is done by a corneal transplant. When I trained, the only way to do that was with a full thickness piece of cornea with its healthy endothelium. In recent years, surgeons have begun to transplant only the posterior layers of the cornea including the endothelium. This tissue is from an eye from someone who has recently died and donated their eye.

See the chapter on corneal transplants for more details.

Retinal detachment after cataract removal

Removing the cataractous human lens from the eye and replacing it with a thin plastic lens changes the fluid dynamics of the eye.

The normal human lens with the supporting zonules, the suspensory ligaments that hold it in place, separates the front of the eye from the back and holds the vitreous back. The implant lens occupies less space and is less stable than the original lens. This allows the vitreous more freedom of movement within the eye. If the vitreous is firmly attached to points on the retina, as it some times is, this vitreous movement may tear the retina and cause a retinal detachment. This happens after less than one percent of cataract operations unless there are complications at surgery such as rupture of the lens capsule and/or loss of vitreous jelly from the eye. The incidence of retinal detachment is nine times higher after such surgical complications.

After the retina begins to detach, the patient notices a shadow or curtain in one part of their vision. This shadow represents the area of detached retina and it may shift or enlarge. Another sign of retinal detachment is light flashes like fireworks and a new crop of floating black dots, called floaters. Either of these signs indicates a medical emergency. The patient should be seen by an ophthalmologist the day it happens or, at the latest, the next day.

Receptionists are trained to respond to complaints of flashes and floaters by arranging immediate access to the doctor.

Treatment may be as simple as injecting an air bubble into the eye to hold the retina in place until it sticks to the surrounding tissue that has been frozen to make it inflamed. It may be as complicated as surgically placing a band around the eye with a small piece of silicone placed outside of the eye over the retinal hole, or tear, to push, or buckle, the outer coats of the eye in toward the hole in the retina to close it. This may be combined with removal of all of the vitreous from the eye and filling the eye with air or a special gas.

If the detachment is discovered and fixed before it has extended to the macula, the center of vision, the chances of retaining good vision are much better than if the detachment has extended into the macular area. The area of detachment tends to spread as time passes so immediate surgery is necessary to stop the spread.

Dropped lens fragments

When I learned to do cataract surgery, we removed the cataract in one piece. The eye was opened with a large incision along the edge of the cornea. This incision extended half way around the cornea. The assistant lifted the free edge of the cornea while the surgeon pulled the iris back with an iris retractor and then put and cold probe onto the front of the lens. The probe was cooled to -60 degrees Centigrade and therefore froze instantly to the lens capsule and front layers of the lens. Withdrawing the probe from the eye while it was frozen to the lens, pulled on the lens, breaking the zonules. The lens could then be slid from the eye.

One of the complications that could occur was the tearing of the capsule. This allowed the nucleus of the lens to drop into the eye and disappear into the vitreous. Before vitreous surgery was possible in the early 1970's, this was a disaster. The nucleus, without a capsule covering it, would cause inflammation that lead to retinal detachment or possibly intractable glaucoma.

Modern cataract surgery uses a small, two to three millimeter incision. The lens capsule is deliberately torn in a large circle so that the lens nucleus can be separated from the outer layers of the lens and either brought forward through the pupil and out of the lens or left in place within the capsule bag. An ultrasound probe is used to chisel the nucleus into tiny fragments that are aspirated from the eye through the small incision. The remaining lens material is aspirated from the eye, emptying the capsule. The implant lens is then placed into the capsule through the hole in the capsule that was made before the nucleus was removed. The capsule then holds the lens in position behind the pupil.

During the removal of the nucleus, there are many stresses on the capsule and the round opening in the capsule may extend to tear the capsule. If this tear extends to the back side of the capsule, parts of the nucleus may drop into the back of the eye.

When this happens, the lens material must be removed from the eye to prevent inflammation. To do this, the vitreous and dropped lens material must be removed. Vitrectomy is usually done by a retina surgeon and should be done within hours or days of the cataract surgery. Vitrectomy to save the eye increases the incidence of retinal detachment in the days following the vitrectomy, but removal prevents the eventual vitreous and retinal retraction that leads to an inoperable total retinal detachment.

Dislocated Implant Lens

One of the challenges that came with placing small plastic lenses in the eye to replace the human lens was being able to keep the lens in position. The first implant lenses were developed by Dr. Harold Ridley in England. Before that it was widely believed that the eye would not tolerate any foreign body. Dr. Ridley had observed airmen from World War II who had small pieces of bomber windshields in their eyes, but had no reaction to the plastic from the windshields. He used that plastic to designed lenses the size, shape and optical power of the human lens that was removed. These lenses were made of Perspex CQ that is a polymethyl methacrylate that had been hardened (totally polymerized) with ultraviolet light.

These lenses were heavy and tended to slip out of position and sometimes wandered within the eye. Smaller, lighter, lenses were developed with the required optical power by Dr. Jan Worst in Holland. These were secured by platinum wire loops that extended through the pupil. Other designs placed the lens in a rectangular or triangular sheet of plastic. The corners of these lenses were placed in the anterior chamber in the angle between the iris and the cornea.

The chairman of department during my residency, Dr. D. DuPont Guerry III, experimented with one of the early models of anterior chamber intraocular lenses. They were too small and moved around within the eye causing inflammation that was detrimental to the eye. These lenses were made of plain PMMA that had not been hardened with ultraviolet light. Dr. Guerry concluded that the eye would not tolerate a plastic lens. We had orders to call Dr. Guerry if we saw a patient with one of these lenses in the clinic. He would drop everything and come to the clinic to talk the patient into having the lens removed before it ruined their eye.

Once the correct length of the lens was established, the lenses were stable. It was also learned that the hardened plastic was also essential to the success of the lens implant. Plastic that was not hardened by UV light would leach monomer that had not polymerized, which was toxic to the eye. New implant lenses contain a chemical that absorbs harmful ultraviolet light to keep it from damaging the retina.

The anterior chamber lenses, which were positioned in front of the pupil, could block the flow of ocular fluid through the pupil causing painful glaucoma. Iridectomy, cutting a hole in the peripheral iris, relieved the blockage by providing a secondary pathway for the fluid to enter the anterior chamber and exit through the trabecular meshwork.

Pupil supported lenses depended on the size of the pupil to hold the lens in place. They could also block the pupil, so a peripheral iridectomy was always performed at the time that the lens was inserted. If the pupil dilated, the wire loops could slip through the pupil, dropping the lens into the front or back of the eye, depending on the position of the patient at the time the pupil dilated. The pupil dilates when a person is tired, is in the dark, is under the influence of alcohol or certain drugs, and during sexual activity.

To treat this dislocation, the pupil was dilated using weak dilator eye drops and the patient was positioned so that the lens would settle into the pupil (face up or face down). Once the lens had settled into position, pilocarpine eye drops were squirted onto the eye to constrict the pupil to capture the lens in the pupil again. The patient was then given low dose pilocarpine to use every six to eight hours to keep the pupil constricted all of the time to prevent subsequent dislocation. Elaborate suturing techniques were developed to stabilize these loose lenses without opening the eye. Once the lens was sutured in place, the pilocarpine drops could be discontinued.

The techniques of cataract extraction have changed. When phacoemulsification was developed, the open capsule bag that remained after the opaque parts of the cataract had been removed became a convenient place to put the implant lens. Once the lenses were put into the capsule bag, the incidence of lens dislocation decreased to a rare event. Sometimes, one of the loops that were supposed the hold the lenses in the center of the bag would slip out of the bag or perhaps it was not placed in the bag at the time of surgery. This allowed the lens to ride up or down and become off center. Depending on when this happened, the lens could be removed and replaced or just repositioned by surgery.

Capsular opacity

A common complication of cataract surgery with an implant lens is clouding of the capsule bag that was left in place to hold the implant lens. The clouding is caused by lens cells that migrated from the equator of the lens and the accumulation of fibrous tissue on the capsule. It is virtually impossible to remove all of these cells during surgery. Weeks after surgery, these cells may migrate to the center of the capsule surface behind the new implant lens and scatter the light coming through the pupil. Fibrin may also collect on the surface of the capsule to add to the clouding.

Lens designs have been altered and surgical techniques have been developed to decrease the incidence of capsule clouding, but it still occurs in up to twenty percent of patients. Young patients have a greater tendency to develop capsular clouding. In children, the capsule is opened at the time of cataract removal, because the capsule will cloud within days to weeks. People who are eighty or ninety years old have a low incidence of capsule clouding.

By the time this clouding has occurred, the implant lens is anchored firmly in place. The front and back layers of the capsule bag collapse around the stabilizing loops of the implant lens and stick together like folding tape over string. The capsule holds the lens so firmly that it is sometimes difficult to remove a lens once this has happened.

In the Third World, one of the ways to treat this problem is to enter the eye with a very thin, very sharp knife through the edge of the cornea so that the knife is in front of the iris. The knife is then passed through the pupil and behind the implant. The point of the knife is used to pierce the capsule and to slice a slit in the capsule, a capsulotomy. The elasticity of the capsule bag pulls the slit open to an oval. The cloudy capsule now has a hole as large as the pupil through which the light passes without distortion.

Placing the knife into the eye risks the complications of dislocating the lens, bleeding from the iris, and infection in the eye.

Shortly after the use of intraocular lenses became popular, the YAG laser was developed. It could be used to pop a small hole in the capsule. By linking a line of small holes, the resulting hole became large enough to give good visual results. The laser does not cut the eyeball or introduce bacteria. With reasonable skill the laser will not hit the iris to cause bleeding. The laser light is delivered in a focused cone shaped beam of light with the energy focused at the apex of the cone. The path that goes through the cornea is large enough that the energy is not concentrated and will not burn the cornea. Beyond the apex of the cone which is the focus point, the light diffuses and is harmless. The point of the energy beam is focused slightly behind the lens and capsule so that the energy will break the capsule, but not damage the lens.

Once the capsule is opened, there is no structure in the opening to hold the cells or fibrin so the capsule opacity will not recur in the open area.

RETINAL DETACHMENT

The retina is a complex layer of tissue that chemically converts light into electronic impulses and sends these impulses to the brain for analysis. It is made of layers of nerves, connecting cells known as neurons, supporting cells, and specialized cells known as rods and cones that do the actual conversion from light to chemicals that stimulate the nerves that transmit the impulse to the brain. Behind the rods and cones is a layer of pigment that absorbs light and helps the rods and cones to recover chemically for the next light impulse.

The retina lines the back of the eye as the film in a camera.

Behind or beneath the retina is a layer of blood vessels and pigment called the choroid. It supplies oxygen and nutrition to the retina and removes waste products. The retina is attached in the front of the eye to the pars plana (posterior flat part of the ciliary body) and in the back of the eye to the optic nerve. When the retina is intact, it is held in place by the vitreous gel that fills the eye.

The retina is like the inner tube of a tire that is held against the inside of the tire by pressure from within. If a hole develops in the retina, the liquid portion of vitreous can pass through the retina, undermining the retina and causing it to become detached from the retinal pigment layer and the underlying choroid. The detachment begins at the hole and spreads from there as the escaping vitreous dissects under the retina.

The retina develops holes from trauma and from thinning of the retina secondary to disease or stretching. Various diseases can cause the retina to thin and develop round holes. Where the vitreous gel attaches to the retina, it may pull on the retina. As we age, the vitreous shrinks and it pulls on the attachments to the retina. This traction either detaches the vitreous from the surface of the retina, or it pulls on the retina until a tear develops. These holes usually tear both directions from the point of attachment to form a "U" shaped, or horseshoe tear.

Traction of the vitreous may tear out a round piece of retina that can be seen floating above the hole in the retina. This is called a floating operculum. Tears may be associated with bleeding.

This bleeding is seen as dark spots that float around in the field of vision. They are called floaters. The operculum is sometimes seen as a floater.

People with myopia (nearsightedness) have elongated eyeballs shaped like an olive with the cornea being the pimento. This stretches the retina and thins it near the front of the eye, causing holes to develop. The elongation of the eyeball adds to the traction of the vitreous on the retina. Both the thinning of the retina and the vitreous tension add to the possibility of a retinal detachment in people with significant myopia.

Once the hole develops and the retina becomes detached around the hole, the detachment spreads away from the hole.

As it dissects back toward the macula, it encroaches on the more central visual area and becomes more noticeable to the patient.

As a general rule, the more posteriorly the detachment spreads toward the macula or center of vision, the harder it is to repair and the less likely that good vision will be preserved or restored.

How can you tell if you have a retinal detachment? There are several telltale signs of a retinal detachment. As the retina detaches, it causes the rods and cones at the edge of the detachment to fire as if they had been stimulated by light. The brain sees sparkling lights, like fireworks in the peripheral vision corresponding to the area of the retina involved. If capillaries in the retina are torn, tiny droplets of blood are scattered in the vitreous. These may appear to the person as a swarm of flies or gnats. Larger blood clots may appear as individual moving dark spots, known as floaters. The onset of new floaters may indicate a retinal detachment.

Flashes and floaters should prompt a detailed examination by an ophthalmologist. This exam of the eye is through a dilated pupil, using the indirect ophthalmoscope. This instrument uses a bright light and head held viewing apparatus along with a large lens held in front of the eye by the ophthalmologist. This allows the doctor to see the retina in three dimensions, all the way to the front edge of the retina. The doctor can see any holes in the retina and determine if they are involved in the retinal detachment. The doctor may press on the outside of the eyeball to indent it so that the far peripheral retina can be seen. Holes that cause retinal detachment may occur in this far peripheral retina.

Flashes may be hard to see in bright light and floaters are hard to see against dark backgrounds and at night. Sometime the first thing that a person notices is a shadow or curtain that obscures part of the visual area. This dark area represents the area of the detached retina. In visual areas where both eyes see, vision from the good eye may fill in the shadow so it is not noticed until something, like a hand or falling hair, covers the good eye. This may delay discovery of the detachment for hours or days.

If you have any of these symptoms, you should contact your ophthalmologist immediately or go to the emergency room so that an ophthalmologist can be found to see you right away. A few hours can make a big difference in the success of the repair of a retinal detachment and preservation of vision.

Simple repair

If the doctor finds a small area of detached retina, especially if it is at the top of the eye, he/she may be able to freeze the outside of the eye with a minus 60 degree Centigrade (carbon dioxide)) or a minus 80 degree C (nitrous oxide) freezing rod called a cryoprobe.

This is applied to the outside of the eye over the detachment to induce inflammation around the leaking hole in the retina. A big air bubble is then injected into the eye to float the retina up against the inflamed area so that the inflammation can seal the hole tightly to the inflamed choroid. This may take several days. You may have to sit and sleep for several days in an odd position so that the bubble will be in the right place to lift and hold the retina against the choroid until the edges of the hole stick to the choroid. Once the hole is closed, the eye will remove the fluid that is detaching the retina allowing the retina to settle back into the proper place. If more than one hole is involved with the detachment, the retina will not lay down until all of the holes are closed. Most retinal surgeons will draw a map of the retina before surgery to find all of the holes and locate them on a map of the retina, noting whether the vitreous is attached to the holes and the relationship to the detachment.

Scleral buckle

If the detached area is large, or the detachment is high above the choroid, the surgeon may have to place a silicone band around the eye to squeeze, or buckle, the sclera and choroid toward the center of the eye so that the choroid can come into contact with the retina to close the hole. The inflammation needed to bind the retina to the choroid may be caused by freezing or cautery burns of the sclera and choroid, or laser burns of the retina shot through the pupil. Many retina surgeons partially fill the eye with air or special gasses (SF6) that absorb slower than air. This holds the retina against the inflamed area to seal the hole.

Vitrectomy

For very large detachments of the retina, the surgeon may have to remove all of the vitreous and fill the eye completely with gas or air. For several days after the surgery, the patient should not fly in airplanes or scuba dive. The lower pressure in flying may cause the bubble to expand, or the elevated pressure of diving may increase the nitrogen content of the bubble, increasing the pressure in the eye. If nitrous oxide is used for anesthesia for the surgery, It may be released from tissues and absorbed by the bubble, increasing the pressure in the eye.

Once the eye is "buckled" by an encircling band, removal of the band may cause the retina to become detached again, so the buckle becomes permanent.

If the macula (central vision) was not detached and the holes are well sealed, vision in the eye is usually good after the surgery, except where the retina was detached. This area may never return to the functional level that was present before the detachment.

People who have diseases that cause retinal detachment in one eye are more prone to detachment in the other eye than are the general population. This calls for periodic complete eye exams of both eyes after one retina has detached. The frequency is determined by the pathology present and the time since the first detachment. The retinal surgeon will determine how frequently these exams should be.

Most retinal surgeons that I have known will claim a good surgical result if they have accomplished what they call "anatomical reattachment." This means that the retina is back in place and stable. This may or may not be associated with a return of good vision. Once the macula has detached, there is usually loss of good central vision, although peripheral vision is retained in the areas that were not detached. Some vision may return to areas that were detached and are now reattached.

After trauma and especially in diabetic patients, a fibrous membrane may form on the retina during the healing process.

This is called an epiretinal membrane or sub retinal membrane depending on which side of the retina it develops. As time passes, this membrane may contract, pulling parts of the retina away from the underlying structures and holding them there under tension.

If the process is extensive, the entire retina may become detached, weeks or months after the injury or repair. Before vitreous surgery was invented in the 1960's, it was usually not repairable and all vision was lost in that eye.

Early in the process of membrane formation and traction, the eye may benefit from removal of the vitreous and peeling of the membranes from the surface of the retina to allow it to lie back down against the choroid. This procedure is called a total vitrectomy and membrane peel. Peeling membranes from the surface is a tedious process that is done under the microscope using micro instruments and it requires great skill so that new holes are not torn in the retina. It is like peeling cellophane tape from tissue paper. Fortunately, many tiny instruments, including scissors, various picks, micro forceps, and mini knives, have been developed to help dissect the membranes from the retina.

The vitreous usually begins to liquefy and shrink at about age seventy, plus or minus five years. Diabetic people, because of the increased ions in their vitreous and changes in osmotic pressure caused by high blood sugar, tend to liquefy the vitreous about ten years earlier. This partially explains the higher incidence of retinal detachments in diabetic people.

GLAUCOMA

I have been asked by many patients, "What, exactly, is glaucoma?" When an ophthalmologist defines glaucoma among his colleagues, it is a complex thing to nail down, but, to a lay person, glaucoma is simply elevated pressure in the eye that causes loss of vision. Normal pressure in the eye is considered to be the equivalent to the pressure exerted by a 12 to 21 millimeter high column of mercury (mm Hg). Blood pressure is measured in the same units, but it normally pulses between 120 mm Hg systolic (peak) blood pressure and 80 mm Hg for diastolic (trough) blood pressure. The normal pressure within the eye is much less that the pressure within the blood vessels inside the eye; therefore, the vessels running on the surface of the retina of do not collapse when blood is flowing through them. Venous pressure is near or below the pressure within the eye. The central retinal vein has the lowest pressure in the vascular system in the eye. It can be seen to pulse if the eye pressure is high or the eye is pressed on while the vein is being viewed.

Some pressure within the eye is good. It keeps the eyeball blown up in its spherical shape and holds the contents on the eye in the correct positions. This pressure is generated by a pump mechanism in the ciliary body near the base of the iris. This pump makes and forces nutrient rich fluid into the eye behind the iris.

This fluid flows around the lens and out through the pupil into the anterior chamber (the space between the iris and the cornea).

From there it flows through a meshwork or sieve that lies in the sclera, between the iris and the cornea. After passing through this sieve, it is collected by a small tube that encircles the cornea called Schlemm's canal. This canal feeds the fluid through aqueous veins into the venous blood vessels around the eye where it mixes with the blood.

If the fluid is pumped into the eye and then leaks out at the same rate, the pressure in the eye remains constant. The level of pressure is determined by the resistance of the meshwork to the flow of fluid. If the resistance increases, more pressure is required to push fluid out of the eye. A new higher pressure is established.

With age, the meshwork, called the trabecular meshwork, may collapse and contract, increasing the pressure in the eye. This pressure is transmitted evenly throughout the eye. In adults, the sclera does not stretch to relieve the pressure.

Technically, in chronic simple glaucoma, the most common form of glaucoma, this elevated pressure is not considered glaucoma unless it is high enough to do damage to the eye or vision.

The pressure necessary to cause damage is different for each person. One person may have damage at a pressure of 23 while another may not have damage until the pressure reaches 25 or 27.

The pressure is applied to the veins and capillaries going to the retina and the nerves that exit the back of the eye that transmit impulses from the retina to the brain.

It is controversial, whether the resulting pressure damage to the fibers of the optic nerve is from vascular compromise and decreased blood flow, or is the pressure on the nerves forcing them against the edge of the hole in the sclera through which the optic nerve passes. The tissue plasma that flows up and down the neurons of the optic nerve may be blocked by the pressure that is crimping the nerve fibers against the sclera thereby killing the nerve fiber.

Either way, the pressure in the eye causes death of the nerve fibers, starting with the ones that service the peripheral vision (side vision). It affects the nerves at the top and bottom of the optic nerve preferentially. The first vision lost is in the periphery and in arcs from the optic nerve above and below the center of vision. The central vision and a small peripheral island are among the last to be affected. In people with two working eyes, the vision in one eye will often fill in the visual defects in the image from the other eye, obscuring the visual defects from the patient.

Types of glaucoma

"How do I know if I have glaucoma?" The answer is that most people don't know that they have glaucoma until it has become advanced, or they are discovered to have glaucoma in a routine eye exam or screening exam at a shopping center or church.

The relatively low pressure increase in primary open angle glaucoma does not cause pain or visual symptoms. Some patients bump into cabinet doors or low branches because they do not see them because they have lost peripheral vision. Glaucoma is called, "The sneak thief of vision," because there are no early symptoms.

> I saw a minister who had completely lost vision in one eye and did not know it, because his glaucoma was slower to develop in his other eye, which saw very well. It was not until he somehow covered his good eye that he noticed that he could not see out of his glaucomatous eye.

Unfortunately, once the vision is lost because of glaucoma, only a small amount of the lost vision can be recovered and then only by prompt and adequate treatment. Once the nerve fiber is dead, it cannot be made functional again. Nerves that are injured, but not dead, can be revived by proper care, so some function can possibly be returned.

Another type of glaucoma seems to be an oxymoron. It is called low tension, or low pressure, glaucoma. These people are very sensitive to ocular pressure and show damage to their vision at pressures considered to be in the normal range. They show the typical cupping of the optic nerve and visual field defects that are seen in chronic simple glaucoma from higher pressures.

Treatment involves lowering the pressure to a level that damage does not occur. This may be 10 or 12 mmHg. Getting the pressure this low may require surgery.

There is another form a glaucoma called acute angle closure (or narrow angle) glaucoma that is much less common than chronic simple glaucoma. This form comes in painful attacks with hazy vision and sometimes nausea and vomiting.

Some people have very little room between the iris and the cornea near the trabecular meshwork. If the pupil dilates, the iris falls forward, blocking the access to the meshwork and the out flow from the eye. Acute treatment of this type of attack is to constrict the pupil to pull the angle open to allow the fluid to flow from the eye.

In one form of acute angle closure glaucoma, the iris is pushed forward in the eye by pressure behind the iris. A mildly dilated pupil may be against the lens so tightly that it blocks the flow of fluid in the eye and the pressure builds up behind the relaxed iris.

The iris falls forward until it covers the trabecular meshwork. This blocks the egress of fluid from the eye. The ciliary body continues to pump fluid into the eye causing the pressure to rise quickly to levels of 45 to 60 mm Hg, or higher. The conjunctiva becomes red and the eye can be very painful to the person having the attack.

The pressure forces ocular fluid into the cornea making the cornea hazy. The patient experiences hazy vision and halos around lights.

The high pressure causes nausea and vomiting in some patients.

> We had a patient who was brought into the eye clinic at St. Francis with mildly red eyes. She had a bottle of tobramycin antibiotic eye drops and a bottle of steroid eye drops.
>
> Her care taker told us that she lived in a nursing home.

Three weeks ago both of her eyes became red, so they took her to an emergency room. The doctor there started her on gentamycin eye drops four times a day and told her to come back in a week. Her eye did not improve by the next week so the doctor started steroid drops, four times a day.

A week later, the eyes were still red so he told her to keep taking the medication. Her care taker insisted that she see an ophthalmologist, so she brought her to the clinic.

Her pupils were slightly dilated and her pressures were 35 and 42. Her angles were closed in both eyes. The iris was against the cornea. She had gone into the chronic phase of an acute angle glaucoma attack. She was almost blind. Her pressures had probably been much higher during the initial days of the attack.

We broke the attack in about one hour and lowered her pressures. We put her on weak pilocarpine eye drops, four times a day to keep her from having another attack. We needed to wait for about two weeks for the eye to recover enough that we could perform laser iridectomies in both eyes to avoid future attacks.

The emergency room doctor probably thought that she had conjunctivitis and treated her accordingly. He probably did not have the equipment to check her ocular pressure to learn that she had glaucoma. When it did not get better immediately he should have referred her to an ophthalmologist.

Instead, he added steroids to calm the eye.

If the pressure becomes higher than capillary blood pressure, (somewhere between arterial and venous blood pressures) the vessels in the eye will begin to collapse, compromising blood flow to the retina causing dimming of vision. Some patients loose all visual perception, even of bright lights. If the attack is broken quickly, with the pressure being lowered to normal, the vision usually returns to pre-attack levels. If the attack persists, the visual loss may be permanent. When intraocular pressure rises above the pressure in the central retinal artery it may close the artery, causing irreversible total blindness in that eye. This is very rare.

Intraocular pressure may also collapse the blood vessels in the iris, decreasing the blood supply to the muscles that dilate and constrict the pupil. This interferes with the primary means of breaking the attack. Breaking the attack involves constricting the pupil to pull the iris away from the meshwork to open the outflow channels. One way of treating a glaucoma attack is to shine a very bright light into the eye. This causes the pupil to constrict.

Paralysis of the pupil muscles from decreased blood flow to them often prevents pupil constriction. Eye drops and oral or intravenous Diamox may be used to decrease production of the fluid and decrease the pressure in the eye to allow blood flow to the iris muscles. Intravenous manitol or urea may be given to draw fluid from the eye and shrink the vitreous to lower the pressure and to allow the iris to fall back, opening the fluid access to the trabecular meshwork.

> I saw three patients during my three years of residency who had been operated on for acute bowel obstruction when their problem was actually an attack of acute angle closure glaucoma. There is physiologic response to the obstruction of any hollow organ in the body, such as the gall bladder, the urinary bladder, the ureters, the intestines, and the eyeball. Acute glaucoma is an obstruction of the eyeball. This response affects the gastrointestinal tract. The bowl function stops, causing a condition known as ileus.
>
> Ileus is the cessation of peristalsis, the rhythmic movement of the bowel necessary for digestion and

evacuation of the bowel. The symptoms, bloating, abdominal pain, nausea, and vomiting are the same as for a bowel obstruction.

This ileus often makes glaucoma treatment difficult because the patient cannot take oral Diamox, because of the nausea and vomiting.

Another mechanism for glaucoma attacks is for the iris to dilate in dim light, allowing the peripheral iris to bunch up in front of the trabecular meshwork, blocking outflow. In this form, the lens does not block the pupil, but outflow is still blocked. The treatment is the sameby constricting the pupil and opening fluid access to the trabecular meshwork.

Although most people think of glaucoma as an adult disease, children can be born with glaucoma which is related to imperfect formation of the outflow channels within the eye. There is a controversial theory that a membrane covers the trabecular meshwork.

Slitting this membrane relieves the glaucoma. Pathologists have been unable to demonstrate this membrane to validate the theory. The surgery splits the trabecular meshwork, perhaps creating a direct pathway to Schlemm's canal.

These children may have cloudy corneas and show an aversion to light such as squinting or burying their face in a blanket or pillow. Infants with glaucoma will fuss when they are in bright light. The clouding of the cornea is from fluid forced into the cornea which can be painful. Sometimes the pressure in the eye will cause the posterior layers of the infant cornea to stretch and split, allowing the fluid in the eye to enter the cornea and cause it to be hazy and painful. If untreated, the eye of a child will stretch, making the cornea, and the whole eye, larger. The eye looks like the eye of a cow, so it is called buphthalmia. Some parents think that the child has big beautiful eyes and do not think that they are abnormal.

Juvenile glaucoma develops in children and teenagers. It is hard to diagnose at this age because it is usually asymptomatic. It slowly damages the optic nerve and obliterates peripheral vision, but causes no pain or other discomfort. It is usually found during an eye exam for myopia or symptomatic hyperopia. There is a campaign to promote measurement of ocular pressure in young people to detect this type of glaucoma in the early stages.

Glaucoma is very rare before the age of thirty; so many eye doctors, in todays rushed environment, do not check the pressure in young people.

> I had a teenaged patient with juvenile glaucoma who was treated with Timoptic (timolol) to decrease the fluid production in her eye. When school started in the fall, she complained that she could not keep up with her high school marching band, because she was out of breath most of the time. Timoptic is a beta blocker that decreases fluid production in the eye. It has a side effect that it diminishes stamina by decreasing, or limiting, the heart rate and the breathing rate. I switched her to other medications that lowered her pressure without interfering with her activities.

Both congenital and juvenile glaucoma are usually treated surgically.

Medical treatment with eye drops may not be effective.

The prospect of a lifetime of eye drops to control the glaucoma is depressing, so surgery is done for these patients to create a leak or artificial channel to lower the pressure. Sometimes medical treatment is needed after surgery to further control childhood glaucoma.

People with chronic inflammation in the eye may have blockage of the outflow channels with inflammatory cells or scarring.

This blockage leads to increased pressure sufficient to cause glaucoma damage. This is known as secondary or inflammatory glaucoma.

Trauma may cause damage to the outflow channels. This may cause a delayed onset glaucoma that develops months to years after the trauma. One form is called angle recession glaucoma in which the fluid in the anterior chamber is displaced laterally by a blow to the eye. It dissects between the cornea and iris, through or near, the trabecular meshwork. This allows the meshwork to collapse and block outflow. People with blunt trauma to the eye should be checked for angle recession several weeks after the trauma using a special lens that allows direct visualization of the angle structures. If recession is present, they should be checked for glaucoma every six months for two years or more from the time of the trauma.

Dislocation of the lens, either from disease such as Marfan's syndrome or from trauma, often causes glaucoma. This form may be refractory to treatment and must be pursued aggressively to prevent blindness. Surgery is often necessary to control the glaucoma.

Treatment of glaucoma

Treatment of glaucoma varies with the type of glaucoma being treated. Chronic simple glaucoma, sometimes known as open angle glaucoma, requires long term treatment and follow up visits for pressure checks and visual field measurement. The various means to measure intraocular pressure do not lend themselves to self measurement by the patient. Therefore the patient must come to the doctor's office for pressure measurements, at least every three months. If the pressure is out of control the measurements must be more frequent while the medications are adjusted to control the pressure.

In the United States, the initial treatment for open angle glaucoma is with eye drops. There are several types of eye drops that lower pressure in different ways. Most doctors have a protocol that they follow as to which drops to use first and which to add if the pressure is not controlled. The goal is to get the pressure within the normal range of 12 to 21 mm Hg. Many doctors try for a lower pressure below 16 or 17 mm Hg.

The optimum goal of treatment is to prevent progression of visual damage. This is measured by testing the area of good vision and looking for blind spots within the visual area. This is called visual field testing. A white dot on a stick moved in front of a dark background, or a light projected into a bowl in front of the patient, is brought in from the side of the patient until the patient says that they see the spot or they press a button to indicate that they have seen the spot. This is done all around the perimeter, from both sides and above and below. The points where the spot is seen are mapped on a chart. Different sizes of dots or different brightness of the light are mapped. Small dots and dimmer light are more sensitive to find subtle defects. Changes in the shape of this visual area and blind spots within the visual area indicate progression of the glaucoma.

The doctor can also tell if there is progression of damage by looking at the optic nerve where it enters the back of the eye. By looking in through the pupil, the doctor can see the damage to the optic nerve fibers by observing the depression in the center of the nerve. The nerves fibers come from the peripheral retina, along the front surface of the retina, to form the optic nerve where they leave the eye. As they turn to leave the eye, they form a funnel shape in the center of the nerve. When damage to the nerves occurs, this funnel enlarges to form a cup. If the damage is severe, the cup in the center of the nerve is ballooned out to form a bean pot shape. The vessels that enter the eye through the center of the optic nerve are pushed to the nasal side of the nerve to the edge of the cup. They may disappear from view until they climb back over the sclera rim to enter the eye. This is called a bean pot cup and it occurs when almost all vision is lost to glaucoma.

The optic nerve fibers within the eye do not have a myelin sheath, so they are clear as they run on the surface of the retina, allowing light to pass through them to the photoreceptors (rods and cones). When a monochromatic light is used in the ophthalmoscope, it creates optical interference patterns in the nerve bundles which can be seen as streaks on the retina. Absence of these streaks indicates the death and disappearance of a nerve bundle which has been damaged from glaucoma. Almost all ophthalmoscopes have a green light, called a red free light, which can be used for that purpose. Very few ophthalmologists use it. They prefer to rely on the visual field and changes in the cup size to determine progression of glaucoma damage.

New computerized cameras can photograph the optic nerve in three dimensions and analyze the cup by computer. They can compare it with images taken on prior visits to determine if there has been a subtle change in the cup. They can also predict where visual field changes have occurred by notches in the wall of the cup.

Medications for Glaucoma

There are several types of eye drops to treat glaucoma. The old standby is Pilocarpine. This drug makes the pupil constrict, pulling on the iris which in turn pulls the trabecular meshwork open.

In angle closure glaucoma, it pulls the iris away from the meshwork, allowing the fluid to leave the eye to lower the pressure.

Pilocarpine drops are used four times a day. It has been largely replaced by drops that are needed only once or twice each day.

Epinephrine-like drugs that affect the sympathetic nervous system decrease the amount of fluid made by the ciliary body and thereby reduce the amount of fluid to elevate the pressure. They can be used with other drops to get better control of the pressure.

Later versions of sympathetic eye drops affect the alpha and beta receptors of the ciliary body to control pressure.

Stimulation of alpha receptors decreases fluid production, so alpha stimulators (agonists) are used to decrease pressure. Alpha agonists can cause dryness of the eyes and mouth, difficulty breathing, low blood pressure and chest pain. People using alpha blockers for urinary retention or other problems may not respond well to alpha agonist treatment for glaucoma. Alphagan (brimonidine) is an alpha agonist. It is usually used twice a day.

Beta blockers (antagonists) like Timoptic (timolol) block the beta stimulation of fluid production, also decreasing the pressure.

It is usually used twice a day, but some people may be controlled with only one drop per eye per day. Timolol may cause difficulty breathing, slow heart rate and low blood pressure. Both alpha agonists and beta blockers can cause or exacerbate depression.

Beta blockers are used to alleviate anxiety and control tremors.

Residents in ophthalmology use it to control minor tremors in the operating room while they are learning eye surgery. One drop under the tongue can decrease nervousness and stop tremors.

> One of my residents had a tremor when he operated. I suggested that he try the timolol trick, but he declined because he jogged every morning and had a resting pulse of about forty beats per minute. He was afraid that the timolol would degrease his heart rate further and he would pass out in the operating room.

Another class of anti-glaucoma, eye drops in the prostaglandin analogs. The three common prostaglandin analogs are Xalatan (latanoprost), Travatan (travoprost) and Lumigan (bimatoprost).

They have the advantage of being used only once per eye per day.

They increase outflow of aqueous from the eye to lower pressure.

One notable side effect is the darkening of the eye lashes and the iris. Patients must be aware of, and agreeable to, this change in their appearance. Bimatoprost in bottled as LatisseR and sold as an eye lash enhancer.

All of these drops that decrease fluid production or increase outflow can be used together (one from each class), if necessary, to get the pressure down to a level that does not cause progression of visual loss. In most cases it is not necessary to use more than one or two types of eye drops. Newer versions of alpha and beta receptor drugs are more specific for the control of intraocular fluid and have fewer systemic side effects from alpha and beta functions in other parts of the body.

When I was in training, Diamox was used to lower ocular pressure. It also causes the kidneys to work overtime, so patients usually do not like to use Diamox. They may have to get up several times during the night to urinate. Another side effect is tingling of the fingers and toes. This is disturbing to the patients.

Diamox also causes impotence and decrease in libido. A patient in Richmond refused to take Diamox because it caused him to "lose his nature," which made his wife complain about his medications.

We still use Diamox occasionally, for one or two doses, to break a stubborn angle closure attack, but not for chronic therapy.

Surgery for Glaucoma

In bad cases of glaucoma, we cannot bring the pressure down with eye drops to the level where there is no further damage to the optic nerve. When this happens, we resort to laser treatment.

Using the laser, fired through a special magnifying gonioscopic mirror lens, we burn spots on the trabecular meshwork. These burn spots shrink the meshwork where they are and stretch the meshwork open between the spots. This often results in better outflow and lower ocular pressure. This treatment lasts for several months to several years but often must be repeated. If half of the trabecular meshwork has been treated and later failed, the other half can be treated to prolong the effect. Some people get such a good response from this procedure that they can stop taking glaucoma eye drops.

Another treatment uses a different type of laser to burn the ridges of the ciliary body where the fluid is made. The higher the pre laser pressure the more ridges must be burned to lower the pressure to a safe level. Burning too many ridges may lower the pressure too much so this treatment may be done is stages.

The laser does not work for some patients so we have to resort to surgery to make a new outflow channel. There have been many operations devised to do this, but the number of operations invented indicates that most of them do not work very well or last very long.

The most popular filter operation today is the trabeculectomy or some variation of it. This is a guarded hole in the sclera that allows fluid to escape slowly from the eye, but still retain sufficient pressure in the eye to keep its shape and function.

To perform a trabeculectomy, the surgeon dissects the conjunctiva from the surface of the eye and reflects it forward toward the cornea, exposing the sclera directly over the trabecular meshwork near the edge of the cornea. A groove, about half the thickness of the sclera, is made to outline a 3 mm by 5mm rectangle on three sides with no grove on the long side along the edge of the cornea. The top half of the sclera within this groove is elevated surgically to make a flap, hinged at the cornea. A small square of the underlying tissue is removed under this flap to extend through the full thickness of the sclera, through the trabecular meshwork. This opens a channel from the inside of the eye into this hole where the square was removed. The flap is then sewn over this hole with two stitches at the corners, leaving the edges loose, to leak slowly. The conjunctiva is then replaced to cover the whole area with the edges of the conjunctival incision sewn together to make a water tight closure.

The next day, the conjunctiva has become ballooned up by the escaping fluid that is trapped beneath it. This creates some pressure in the eye that is usually in the low normal range. If it is too high, we use the laser, through the conjunctiva, to cut one stitch, releasing one corner. This reduces the pressure further. If necessary the second stitch can be cut with the laser at a later procedure to further decrease the pressure.

There are many variations on this procedure to create a leak to lower the pressure.

When I was in Galveston, we had a large population of black patients with uncontrolled glaucoma who needed surgery. One of our faculty members, Dr. R. Michael Nisbet, had just come from Detroit where the cyclodialysis procedure was popular. He claimed that it worked well in black patients. We set up a study in which half of the patients, either black or white, had the popular trabeculectomy procedure and half had the cyclodialysis procedure.

Patients were matched randomly to procedures. This was considered ethical because the effectiveness of each procedure in the two races had not been established.

After a year we evaluated the results and found that our success rate for trabeculectomy was much better in white patients.

However, the success rate for trabeculectomy was very poor in black patients. The cyclodialysis procedure worked very well in black patients, so thereafter we used the best procedure for each group. In complicated cases it was sometimes necessary to do both procedures if the first one failed.

In the cyclodialysis procedure, the conjunctiva is opened parallel to the nasal side or the superior rectus muscle (the muscle at the top of the eye that moves the eye upward). The muscle was grabbed with a forceps and pulled to one side. A full thickness incision was made through the sclera immediately behind and beneath the attachment of the muscle, parallel to the edge of the cornea. A special blunt needle spatula (curved hollow spatula) was introduced into the incision and pushed forward between the sclera and the choroid until the tip broke through to the anterior chamber and could be seen through the cornea. This spatula was swept from side to side, detaching the iris root and ciliary body from the sclera and disrupting the blood supply to the ciliary body in that area. An air bubble was injected through the spatula needle to fill the cleft made by the spatula between the sclera and ciliary body to hold it open for several days. Once the bubble was in position, the spatula was removed and the muscle was released; closing the incision. The conjunctiva was then closed with sutures. The patient was asked to sit up on the operating table to be sure that the bubble went into the cleft. They slept on several pillows to be sure that the bubble stayed in the cleft.

After several days, the bubble was absorbed and the cleft healed as an open passage, allowing ocular fluid to flow back between the sclera and choroid where it was reabsorbed by the choroid. The tension on the zonules, (the threads from the ciliary body to the lens that hold the lens in place), pull the cleft open.

This procedure does not work as well in people who have had the cataract removed in that eye, because the tension on the zonules is diminished or absent. Cyclodialysis works very well in black patients who have not had a cataract removed.

Many procedures have been tried to place a seton, a tube or rod, through the sclera, extending between the anterior chamber of the eye and the space between the sclera and the conjunctiva, to make a permanent drain. If this is a hollow tube, the fluid drains out and the eye collapses. A solid rod will create a leak, like a nail in a tire, but it will eventually encapsulate or seal off so that the fluid stops flowing. In recent years, tubes have been developed with valves that create enough resistance to keep the eye inflated while allowing sufficient leak to relieve excess pressure.

Some tubes with valves are made that end in reservoir that allows the fluid to slowly leak under the conjunctiva to be absorbed.

These are usually the last resort in treating glaucoma, but they are effective.

One other treatment that has fallen into disfavor, because of the pain and swelling that lasts for a week or more, is called cyclo-cryo therapy, meaning that the ciliary body (cyclo) is frozen (cryo). In this treatment, a cryoprobe is placed over the conjunctiva and sclera in the area over the ciliary body. The temperature of the cryoprobe is reduced to—60 (carbon dioxide probe) or—80 (liquid nitrogen probe) degrees centigrade and kept there for twenty or thirty seconds. The probe is allowed to thaw and then frozen for another period. The ice ball formed within the eye damages the ciliary body reducing the production of fluid. Multiple sites are frozen, sparing the areas near the muscle attachments, so the arteries to the front of the eye are not damaged. The pressure in the eye is measured every week for the next month. Usually the pressure drops to below normal in the first few days and slowly rises back into the normal range by one month after the treatment. The final pressure at one month is used to determine whether another treatment is necessary and, if so, how much area to retreat. Over treatment may make the eye collapse and go blind, a condition known as phthisis bulbi (tie sis bull buy). Protocols, relating preoperative pressure to treatment area and time of freeze, have been developed to treat and retreat without ruining the eye.

Chronic simple glaucoma is treated, not cured. It is a lifelong disease once it has occurred. In the majority of cases it can be controlled by eye drops. Only progressive cases must be treated by laser or surgery. In Europe and many other parts of the world, the treatment philosophy is different. Many ophthalmologists there operate first and when that eventually fails; they either reoperate or change to eye drops. In parts of the world where eye drops are hard to obtain, surgery may be the best treatment. When there are no ophthalmologists to do the surgery, doctors and nurses use the drops. Unfortunately, in some parts of the world, there is neither eye drops nor surgeons to do the surgery to treat glaucoma.

During the weeks after glaucoma surgery, the pressure can change and it may take several months to stabilize. During that time, the surgeon may need to do several procedures to lower the pressure, if it is still too high. On our trips to the Island of Montserrat to provide eye care, we did not do glaucoma surgery because there were no doctors there to do those adjustments that might be needed, after we left. Eye drops were a more reliable means of treatment and could be regulated by the trained ophthalmic nurse, using a flow scheme that we had taught her.

I recently attended a meeting where a new glaucoma treatment was introduced. This involved tiny tubes with a tiny blade that stuck out at right angles to the tube. These are placed in the trabecular meshwork from the inside of the eye during cataract surgery to create new pathways for the fluid to exit the eye. The inventors claimed excellent results in treating cataract patients who had glaucoma. These tubes are still experimental.

> I had an eighty-two-year-old woman patient, a doctor's widow, who went to Afghanistan with an aid group during the invasion by Russia. I gave her a prescription for her eye drops for enough medication to last her a year. I saw her in my office about a year later when she needed more drops.
>
> She told me that glaucoma medications were not available anywhere in Afghanistan.
>
> She told me that she and several other members of her group had gotten out of Afghanistan just in time when Russia pulled out and left Afghanistan to the Taliban.
>
> Some of her coworkers were captured and were still being detained. She took up volunteering at Meals on Wheels since she could not go back to Afghanistan.

The exception in treating glaucoma for a cure is in cases of angle closure glaucoma. Since the cause of angle closure glaucoma is mechanical, with the iris being pushed forward to block the outflow pathways, the cure is also mechanical. By making a hole in the iris near the outer edge or base of the iris, the ocular fluid is allowed to flow directly from the posterior chamber, behind the iris, into the anterior chamber, in front of the iris. This hole equalizes the pressure on the iris and prevents the fluid from pushing the iris forward to block the outflow paths.

When I trained, this hole, called an iridectomy, was made by cutting into the eye at the edge of the cornea and allowing the iris to prolapse from the eye through the small incision. A small piece of the iris was cut away, being sure that the hole was through the full thickness of the iris. The cut piece of the iris was rubbed on the surgical drape. If it left black pigment on the drape we knew that the hole was full thickness because the pigment is on the back of the iris. The prolapsed iris was then milked back into the eye by stroking the cornea, so no instrument actually entered the eye. A single stitch was used to close the incision. From that day onward, a triangular hole could be seen at the outer edge of the iris. The hole did not heal and close.

> When I was a fellow at the Massachusetts Eye and Ear Infirmary, I was able to watch Dr. Paul Chandler, one of the icons of glaucoma therapy, perform a peripheral iridectomy.
>
> He had done so many that it only took him about two minutes to do the whole procedure, once the eye was prepped and draped. When students came to the operating room to watch, he often sent them to get the operating room supervisor just as he was about the make the scleral incision. By the time they returned, he had finished the procedure. He did this to emphasize the short duration of the procedure. If the student was smart, they were not fooled a second time.

With the advent of the xenon arc photo coagulator, it was possible to burn a hole through the iris using repeated burns, without making an incision. We now use the argon laser which is more efficient and less likely to damage the cornea. When the laser has burned all the way through the iris, a small cloud of pigment from the back surface of the iris flows through the hole. This proves that the hole is all the way through the iris. In many offices, the argon laser has now been replaced by the YAG laser which blasts a hole through the iris in one or two multishot pulses.

Many people will develop a cataract in the eye that has received an iridectomy several years after the surgery. This was usually blamed on the surgeon having inadvertently touched the lens in the eye with an instrument when the hole was cut in the iris. In the new surgical techniques, no instruments enter the eye, yet cataracts develop. Cataracts still develop after laser surgery where no instruments are introduced into the eye to possibly touch the lens.

My theory of the cause is based on nutrition of the lens. The intraocular fluid contains nutrients and free radical scavengers that retard cataract formation. I believe that the change in flow of the fluid through the iridectomy from behind the iris to the front of the iris, without bathing the lens in nutrients and radical scavengers, as it would going through the pupil, causes the lens to age prematurely. Research has shown that free radicals play a role in preventing cataract formation.

Other Medications and Glaucoma

People who have glaucoma often encounter directions on a medication that they take, telling them that they should not take the medicine if they have glaucoma. When I worked at the U.S. Food and Drug Administration, I was assigned to follow the drugs ValiumR and LibriumR. They were already on the market, but the company that made them wanted this restriction for glaucoma to be removed from the label or relaxed in some way.

Both LibriumR and ValiumR caused the pupil in the eye to dilate slightly. The original reviewers were afraid that this pupillary dilation might precipitate an angle closure glaucoma attack, so they put in the restriction that these drugs should not be taken if the patient had glaucoma. They were not ophthalmologists and did not discriminate between chronic simple, (open angle) glaucoma and angle closure glaucoma. Chronic simple glaucoma is much more common than angle closure glaucoma. Only the angle closure patients needed to worry.

Many patients with chronic simple glaucoma were taking one or the other of these drugs, not knowing that the printed label warned against taking them. They did not have complications with their glaucoma. Patients who know that they have open angle glaucoma or angle closure glaucoma and are being treated for it have no trouble taking either ValiumR or LibriumR while their glaucoma is being treated.

The people who can get in trouble are the ones with narrow angles who do not know that they have them. If the pupil dilates, the angle could be compromised and cause a glaucoma attack.

If the narrow angle has been diagnosed and treated with either weak pilocarpine drops or a peripheral iridectomy (hole in the iris), the angle will not close when the pupil dilates slightly from the medication, so they can also safely take the medications.

My job was to develop a wording that could convey this correctly.

The people at risk were people who had narrow angle glaucoma, but did not know it. I wrote a memorandum to the commissioner's office explaining the situation and they replied that they would try to work out some wording that conveyed that concept. It did not happen while I was at the FDA, but I think the final wording was that people who had "uncontrolled glaucoma" should not take these drugs. This wording still does not help the people who do not know they have narrow angles. If you are taking any of these drugs, you should ask your eye doctor whether you have a risk of glaucoma *attacks*. Your ophthalmologist can check your angles and tell you.

There are many drugs that affect the pupil by dilating or constricting it. Either movement of the pupil can precipitate a glaucoma attack, so all of these drugs have the caveat about uncontrolled glaucoma.

CORNEAL TRANSPLANTS

There are many eye diseases that affect the cornea and cause it to lose the function of a clear optical lens. The cornea is made of long collagen fibers that run in parallel bundles from one side of the cornea to the other. The space between the fibers is filled with a clear viscous material, a glycose aminoglycan, which makes the cornea optically clear. When I went to medical school, glycose aminoglycans were known as mucopolysaccharides.

My German biochemistry professor loved to pronounce mucopolysaccharide.

When the regular pattern of the fibers is disrupted, or the surface of the cornea becomes irregular from trauma or disease, the optical properties are destroyed. Light is blocked or scattered and cannot form a clear image on the retina.

Metabolic diseases of the cornea are caused by absence of one or more enzymes that help to break down damaged tissue or metabolic waste products so that they can be removed from the cornea. These diseases are called hereditary dystrophies. Some are transmitted as dominant genetic traits and some are recessive.

The recessive dystrophies may skip generations.

The metabolic waste products collect in the cornea as white dots, lines or ridges. They collect in distinctive patterns—superficial, deep, central, peripheral, sharp edged, fuzzy edged, comma shaped, etc. Doctors who describe a new pattern or shape usually have that pattern named for them. There are many named dystrophies, but my mentor, Dr. Claes Dohlman, once told me, "there are actually two kinds of dystrophies: those that interfere with vision and need to be operated and those that do not interfere with vision and should be left alone." Actually, knowing the appearance and cause of the dystrophy allows us to know how it will behave and when it may deteriorate.

There is a belief among corneal surgeons that to become The Professor at a European eye institute, the doctor had to have a corneal dystrophy named after him. This is what led to the hair splitting of details about dystrophies: about the shape and distribution of the corneal opacities, i.e. dots, spots, commas, circles, single lines, horse tail lines, deep, superficial, central, peripheral, sharp edged, wooly, etc.

Some dystrophies interfere with vision at a young age. These include congenital cloudy cornea, granular dystrophy, macular dystrophy, lattice dystrophy (including Reis-Bucklers dystrophy) and keratoconus. People with these dystrophies usually need to have a corneal transplant by the time they are twenty to twenty-five years old. Some people with granular dystrophy may retain useful vision longer than the other dystrophies. Because the hereditary enzyme defect is not repaired, the corneal opacity may recur in the transplant for some dystrophies.

> When I was in fellowship training at Massachusetts Eye and Ear Infirmary in Boston, a baby was brought to the clinic with white corneas in both eyes. He had been born with cloudy corneas. His father had cloudy corneas that had never been operated. The family told us that the white corneas were a curse from God, because the baby's grandfather had been a wicked man. They quoted the bible saying that, "The sins of the father are vested on the children from generation to generation." The child had congenital corneal dystrophy which is present at birth. Dr. Dohlman and the social service obtained a court order

to operate on this child to do a cornea transplant so the child could see.

About six months after the transplant, the child was brought in with a white spot in the operated cornea, growing from one of his sutures. Culture of that spot grew Nocardia fungus. The steroid drops that were used to prevent rejection of the transplant had allowed the fungus to grow. The antibiotic drops being given to the baby suppressed the bacterial competition and did not inhibit fungal growth.

All of the available antifungal medications were prohibited by the FDA for use in children, so we needed to find another way to treat the fungal infection to save the transplant. I was assigned to research this and find a treatment we could use. I discovered that the method used before antifungal medications were developed was to apply eye drops of super saturated potassium iodide. The pharmacy put potassium iodide crystals in artificial tears and heated them until the solution was super saturated when it cooled. We could tell from the response of the child that the eye drops stung for a few minutes every time they were used, but the spot disappeared in about five days.

This was as fast as we could expect from the common antifungals used in an adult. Some of the old cures still work and are still needed.

Another hereditary dystrophy affects vision in older people.

Fuch's dystrophy is named after the Viennese ophthalmologist, Ernest Fuchs, who first described it. This dystrophy involves the posterior layers of the cornea. Descemet's membrane, the membrane on the back of the cornea that holds the endothelium, develops excrescences, bumps, on the posterior side, called guttata.

They appear like tiny dew drops on the back of the cornea when viewed with high magnification. These bumps disrupt the attached endothelial layer allowing ocular fluid to leak into the cornea, causing the cornea to swell and form blisters under the epithelium. The swelling and the blister bumps blur the vision.

The endothelium is a layer of cells that lie behind Descemet's membrane that form a barrier to keep fluid that is within the eye from entering the cornea. Some intraocular fluid normally leaks into the cornea to transport nutrients to the cornea. This fluid is then pumped back into the eye by the endothelium. Loss of endothelial cells allows more fluid to leak into the cornea and leaves fewer cells to pump fluid back out of the cornea and into the eye. The result is fluid collecting in the cornea, called primary corneal edema. The endothelium does not grow after the first two or three years of life. Therefore the endothelium is not replaced if it is lost by disease or is damaged. To correct the edema problem the sick endothelial layer must be replaced by transplantation of donor tissue.

Damage to the endothelium can also occur from external trauma to the eye or from damage by surgical instruments, intraocular lenses, or irrigation fluids.

A common hereditary corneal problem that occurs before the age of thirty is keratoconus. In keratoconus the center of the cornea becomes thin enough that the pressure in the eye pushes it forward and it sags down. The cornea is usually normal in appearance, but the deformity is sufficient to cause severe myopia and astigmatism by optical changes in the cornea.

Keratoconus is associated with a number of diseases including atopic dermatitis, Marfan's syndrome, Down's syndrome, retinitis pigmentosa, and aniridia.

In the early stages, keratoconus can be treated with hard contact lenses. Eventually, many keratoconus patients progress so that the cornea is somewhat pointed and a contact lens will not stay on the cornea. Picture a hub cap on a traffic cone. Techniques are being developed to shrink the cornea with heat or by inducing cross linking of the collagen fibers to bring back a normal contour of the cornea. The mainstay of treatment of keratoconus is still the corneal transplant, either full thickness (penetrating keratoplasty) or partial thickness (lamellar transplant). Keratoconus has a success rate for a clear, visually successful transplant of about 90-95%

When I was a resident at Medical College of Virginia (MCV), there was a journal article by Dr. David Cogan, the Chairman of Ophthalmology at Harvard Medical School, describing a new corneal dystrophy. This was a superficial dystrophy comprised of clear microcysts beneath the epithelium, near the center of the cornea. He reported several cases. Dr. D. DuPont Guerry, III, our Chairman of Ophthalmology at MCV, told us that he had also discovered these microcysts and was collecting a series. He actually had several more than Dr. Cogan had reported. Dr. Guerry's cases also had, in addition to the cysts, very fine lines that were very superficial, probably just below the epithelium at the same level as the cysts.

Dr. Guerry wrote a letter to the editor of the journal, complimenting Dr. Cogan on his discovery of these cysts in the central cornea. He went on to mention that if Dr. Cogan would widen the beam of light on his slit lamp, (the optical instrument used to examine the cornea), that he would probably find that his patients also had the lines that Dr. Guerry had found. This was a "got ja" in the medical literature. Dr. Guerry and Dr. Cogan were long time friends, but also competitors.

This dystrophy is known as Cogan's dystrophy everywhere except Richmond, Virginia where it is known as Cogan/Guerry dystrophy. Over the years the lines have been described as beach lines, (multiple wavy parallel lines like those made by waves on a beach), mare's tail lines, (a sweep of lines spreading from a point), straight, and wavy lines. They represent folds in the basement membrane between the epithelium and Bowman's layer at the front of the cornea. The cysts are cellular debris trapped under the basement membrane. The same patterns are seen after recurrent erosions of the cornea. Some experts question whether this is a dystrophy or is the left over signs of recurrent erosions. The dystrophy cysts usually do not interfere with vision and are not painful. Recurrent erosions are usually painful.

A number of acquired diseases end with corneal scarring that blocks vision. Corneal ulcers from bacteria, fungus, and viruses all may end in opacity and irregularity of the surface of the cornea.

Diseases like Stevens Johnson syndrome, ocular pemphigoid, Vitamin A deficiency, severe dry eye disease and chemical or thermal burns can all lead to severe scarring that requires a corneal transplant. Most of this last group has a poor prognosis of less than a 50% chance for a long term clear corneal transplant, because the cornea is vascularized and the surface tissues are damaged.

Because of epithelial healing problems in these diseases, we usually do not remove the epithelium from the transplanted tissue and try to get it to survive the transplant procedure. These cases would probably do better with an artificial cornea called a keratoprosthesis.

Keratoprostheses are still relatively experimental. I have spent eighteen years in research to develop a new design for a keratoprosthesis.

Because of FDA requirements, research cannot go to human trials unless there is a corporate sponsor with corporate liability insurance. Requirements for FDA approval make it too expensive for U.S. companies that make similar ocular devices, to produce the new keratoprosthesis, because so few people in the U.S. would need prostheses each year.

Less than five hundred people in the United States need a keratoprosthesis each year and only a fraction of that number actually receives one. UNESCO has determined that about eight million people in the world have blindness secondary to corneal disease and would benefit from an artificial cornea, a keratoprosthesis.

Most of these people are in the third world, so the surgery and maintenance of the keratoprosthesis would have to be simple and straight forward and inexpensive. My prosthesis meets all of these criteria.

Types of corneal transplants

One of the earliest forms of successful corneal transplant is called an anterior lamellar keratoplasty. This transplant uses a donor cornea that is cut to about half thickness using a round circular blade like a biscuit cutter, only much smaller and sharper. The front half of the cornea is then peeled off of the remaining cornea to use for donor tissue. The same circular blade, called a trephine, is used to remove a similar part of the diseased cornea. The new tissue is sewn onto the cornea in the place of the damaged cornea.

This works when the opacity is in the front half of the cornea or in keratoconus where the central corneal must be made thicker.

If the scar or other opacity is too deep in the cornea, the lamellar cornea will not make the cornea clear.

A new procedure, called deep anterior lamellar keratoplasty, replaces almost the full thickness of the cornea, but preserves the recipient's Descemet's membrane and endothelium. It is being used in keratoconus. This has the advantage of decreasing the incidence of immune rejection of the transplant, because the rejection is usually directed at foreign endothelium. In this procedure the patient retains their own endothelium which the body does not try to reject.

When the problem involves the endothelium or the full thickness of the cornea, a full thickness corneal transplant (penetrating keratoplasty) is necessary. The corneal endothelium is only one cell thick which makes it very sensitive to injury. It must never be touched during surgery. The easiest way to transport the corneal endothelium from the donor to the recipient is with it attached to the full thickness button of tissue. The main drawback of this procedure is that the recipient may try to reject the cellular components of the donor cornea.

The normal cornea does not have blood vessels. Keratoconus, Fuch's and other dystrophies, and some corneal ulcers, do not have blood vessels. White blood cells are the major mechanism of sensitization of the body to foreign tissue and for subsequent destruction of the foreign tissue. Although they may wander through the tissues, most white blood cells are in, or near, the blood vessels. Lack of vessels in the cornea makes the cornea a privileged recipient site for donor tissue. The new tissue may be placed in the cornea and the body may not discover that it is foreign tissue and will not reject it. Once the cornea has developed blood vessels in the process of healing an ulcer or burn, the donor tissue does not have this privilege. The body may reject the epithelium, the cells in the stroma (keratocytes), and the endothelium.

The most serious rejection is of the endothelium which cannot regenerate. Once it is rejected, the cornea will remain cloudy, but usually does not dissolve or fall out.

There has been some excitement recently about progress in transplanting a layer of endothelial cells onto the back of the cornea. Some studies have cultured endothelial cells onto permeable membranes and then placed the membrane and culture onto the back of the cornea to replace the sick endothelium. Other surgeons peel a round disk of Descemet's membrane, with the endothelium attached, from the back of a donor cornea and then transplant it onto the back of the patient's cornea. The tissue can be rolled up and injected through a large needle into the front of the eye where it is unrolled. The new layer is held in position by an air bubble or a pillow of viscoelastic material which will later dissolve and be removed from the eye. There have been reports of success with these procedures, but they are still considered to be experimental.

Once donor tissue from another person is transplanted, there will always be the possibility of rejection of the tissue by the body.

If white blood cells are sensitized to the foreign tissue and travel to a lymph node, other white blood cells are sensitized and spread through the body looking for the foreign tissue. White blood cells will attack and kill the foreign cells. They travel through the aqueous fluid and attack the endothelial cells. A line of cells can be seen moving across the corneal endothelium. Once the endothelial cells are dead, the fluid leaks into the cornea and the cornea swells and becomes cloudy.

Cortical steroids can stop this attack and save the corneal endothelium if the rejection is caught in the early stages. Steroids are given as eye drops, injections around the eye and by mouth, to stop the rejection at different levels of the process. Rejection episodes may recur from time to time and may eventually destroy the transplant. After the transplant, use of steroid eye drops, once or twice a day, may prevent rejection or lengthen the time between rejection episodes. Other anti rejection medications from other types of organ transplants are being tried. One that appears to have some success is Cyclosporin A which is now available in eye drop form.

Corneal transplant surgery

Corneal transplants require live donor tissue from a deceased donor. General awareness of the need for transplant tissue has greatly improved in recent years. Vision in both eyes is so important that living donors are not considered unless there is a very unusual circumstance where the donor is blind in the donor eye but the cornea is normal. The donor tissue from the blind eye is replaced with a substandard cornea since vision is not expected.

The tissue from the blind eye is transplanted into the person with the bad cornea. This is an extremely rare situation.

When I did my first corneal transplant in 1970, the eye bank had to wait until someone, who had agreed to donate their eyes, had died; or their next of kin had agreed to donate the eyes of the deceased. A technician or an ophthalmology resident was dispatched to retrieve the donated eyes. The eyes were placed in bottles with wet gauze to keep them from drying out and then refrigerated. Cooling the tissue slowed the metabolism of the cells and preserved the glycogen stores in the cells. As long as there is glycogen for energy, the cell will remain viable and the tissue can be transplanted. The technician would check the hospital chart for evidence that the patient had syphilis, tuberculosis, or hepatitis that would make the eyes unusable.

> Once the eyes were in the eye bank, the eye bank would call the next two surgeons on the list to tell them that tissue was available.
>
> Once notified, I called my patient to tell him to come to the hospital immediately. The patient had been alerted that he was next on the list so he should be waiting with a suitcase packed and a full gas tank. Unfortunately, my first transplant patient did not have a telephone or transportation, so we had to send the sheriff out to get him and bring him to Richmond. Corneal transplants were not very common at that time so the sheriff was happy to assist in bringing the patient ninety miles to the hospital for his surgery.

Tissue was considered viable (active metabolism was still present in the cells) for twenty-four hours. Surgery usually had to be done at night. Tomorrow's operating schedule was set and could not be bumped. Spill over from the day schedule and other earlier emergencies filled the early evening schedule and transplants were added after them. Because of the twenty-four hour time constraint, the tissue would not be usable by the end of tomorrow's schedule.

Progress has changed all of that. The tissue still comes from a recently deceased donor. The corneas with rims of sclera, not the whole eyes, are harvested and immediately placed in a special culture medium that nourishes the tissue and does not allow the cornea to swell. The corneas are checked by a technician for suitability for transplant, including a count of the endothelial cells per square millimeter, and then they are refrigerated. Because of the tissue culture medium and the cooling, corneas can be used for up to five days for a full thickness transplant (penetrating keratoplasty) or several weeks for an anterior lamellar transplant if the epithelium is not critical to the success of the transplant. The recipient will grow epithelium to cover the newly transplanted tissue with their own corneal epithelium in many situations.

Donor epithelium should be transplanted in healthy condition in cases involving herpes scars, chemical burns, and diseases like Stevens Johnson syndrome and ocular pemphigoid to avoid healing problems with the recipient's epithelium.

In modern tissue banking, the medical history of the donor is reviewed and blood, drawn from the donor, is tested for any transmittable diseases such as syphilis, AIDS, or hepatitis. Tissue is not approved for transplant until this review is complete. The chart is reviewed for rare transmittable diseases like Creutzfeldt-Jacob disease or tissue damaging disease like diabetes.

For a while, it was thought that growing the cornea in tissue culture for three weeks or more would prevent immune rejection of the tissue, but that turned out to be a hoax, perpetrated by a zealous researcher doing studies on skin grafts in animals.

His initial results of immune response diminution could not be replicated, so he painted the skin of the white rats black to simulate a black on white skin transplant. The discovery of this deceit prompted many conferences at medical schools across the country on the topic of ethics in research.

Now, eye banks usually have a supply of viable donor corneas on hand at any given time. The doctor schedules surgery at a time that is convenient for both himself and the patient and calls the eye bank to request tissue for that date. The day before the scheduled transplant, the eye bank technician calls the doctor and tells them what corneas are available and then faxes the information about the condition of each available cornea. The doctor evaluates the possible tissue and then chooses the donor cornea that best matches the recipient and then requests that the tissue be delivered to the operating room in time for the surgery. In Houston, or Pittsburgh, I rarely had to cancel and reschedule surgery because there were no corneas available.

> When I lived in Texas, the Houston "Eyes of Texas" Eye Bank usually had extra tissue left in their refrigerator at the end of the week. The eye bank director would put it in a Styrofoam tissue transport box with dry ice and take it to the airport to put it on TWA flight one—The TWA flight that went around the world. That flight stopped in Riyadh, Saudi Arabia, where Dr. David Payton, who had been chairman of Ophthalmology at Baylor Medical School in Houston, was now running the King Kahlid Eye Specialist Hospital. The eye bank would have sent a wire to him to tell him the number of corneas to expect. He would call in that many waiting patients for surgery on Monday. Corneal blindness was common in Saudi Arabia, causing a demand for transplantable corneas.

Transplant procedure

Corneal transplants require the sterile environment of an operating room, either in a hospital or outpatient surgical center. Most facilities require laboratory work to clear you for the surgery that is usually done under local block anesthesia with monitored conscious sedation anesthesia. Conscious sedation means that you may be asleep, but you can be aroused to cooperate if necessary.

Surgery on children and very nervous or incompetent adults is done under general anesthesia.

The nurses that check you in will examine the orders and the chart to determine which eye is to be operated. The eye will be marked, usually by the surgeon, with indelible ink, so the marking will not wash off during the prepping of the surgical area.

Some hospitals require the surgeon to mark the operative site before you can be taken to the operating room

Once in the operating room, the nurses there will check again to be sure they have the correct eye prepped. An anesthesiologist will start an intravenous line and give some relaxing medication.

Some hospitals require a "time out" to be called at this point. All work is stopped so that everyone in the operating room can agree which eye is to be operated and that the correct eye has been prepared for surgery.

The surgeon will anesthetize the eye and further prepare it for surgery. The microscope is moved into place and adjusted by the surgeon so that your eye is in focus and centered in the microscope field and that the magnification is correct. Adjustments can be made by use of a foot pedal during surgery.

A speculum is placed in the eye to hold the eyelids open.

The eye is inspected and irrigated with balanced salt solution to clean the surface and remove any lashes or other debris from the conjunctiva.

If you have had a cataract removed, the surgeon may sew a ring to the front of the eye to keep it from collapsing when the eye is opened. Then the cornea is cut with the round trephine to a depth of about two thirds of the full thickness. Great care is exercised to center the trephine on the cornea to align it with the optical pathway. The trephine is rotated to make it cut into the cornea. The incision is inspected and modified, if necessary. The eye is covered with a moist sponge to keep it wet while the donor tissue is prepared.

The surgeon then takes the donor cornea from the bottle of tissue culture and places it on a cornea block on the side table, endothelium side up. Using the same trephine, or one slightly larger or smaller depending on the disease being treated and technique being used, a full thickness button of tissue is punched from the center of the donor cornea. Care must be taken to avoid touching the endothelium of the donor tissue, except where the blade cuts through it. Simply touching the endothelium may damage it, compromising the survival of the transplanted tissue. This button is moistened with saline or culture medium and placed on the cornea block, under a cover, for safe keeping.

Attention is returned to the recipient eye. The grove that was made with the trephine is now deepened with an ultra sharp knife until the anterior chamber is entered and fluid escapes from the eye. This opening must be large enough to admit the tip of the corneal scissors. Special tiny, curved corneal scissors, right cutting or left cutting, are used to cut the round button free from the cornea along the trephined groove. The button of tissue is then passed to the nurse who will send it to pathology.

The surgeon takes the new cornea from the corneal block and places it endothelial side down in the hole made in the recipient cornea. The button is then sewn in to the cornea with single stitches at twelve, six, three, and nine o'clock to stabilize the new cornea in place and close the eye. Some surgeons continue to put a total of sixteen single sutures. I prefer to use a very fine nylon suture (10-O) on a tiny needle to do a running hem stitch all around the incision line, tying the suture to itself to complete the circle.

I tiny cannula needle is passed through the incision to inject physiologic saline solution into the eye to deepen the space between the new cornea and the iris. The iris is checked to be sure that it was not caught in the incision line and the incision line is checked for leaks. Additional stitches may be placed to stop any leak that is found.

Some surgeons inject antibiotics and steroids in the conjunctiva before closing the eye and putting a patch on the eye to protect it until the anesthetic wears off and eyelid movement is restored.

The surgeon will want to see the patient the next day to check for wound leaks and signs of infection. It may be several days until the cornea recovers full clarity from being refrigerated in the culture media. If one or more sutures are tight, the corneal will be distorted until the tight stitches are removed and vision may not be what was anticipated. The running stitch will usually adjust the tension and the four interrupted stitches can be removed after one or two weeks. If they are tight, the cornea quickly adjusts to the even tension of the running suture. Vision returns faster, in my hands, with the running stitch rather than all interrupted or individual stitches.

Most surgeons will restrict the patient's activity after surgery.

No lifting, no bending at the waist, no driving and no sex for three weeks. I used to be surprised by the number of complaints I received from my older patients about that last restriction.

I have the patient wear a hard plastic or aluminum eye shield over the eye whenever they are not wearing glasses for the first three months. This includes while sleeping. A patient may rub the eye while they are asleep and rupture the fine suture that was used to sew the transplant into the cornea. The patient cannot be responsible for what they do while they are asleep. I'm told that the eye often itches for several weeks after surgery, prompting the patient to want to rub their eye. I think the shield has saved many eyes.

Because there are few or no blood vessels in the cornea it is very slow to heal. I always left the running stitch in place until one year after surgery or until there was a white line in the incision area all the way around the incision. If vision was improved by glasses after three weeks, I usually fit the patient with temporary glasses, knowing that the wound would shift and the glasses would need to be changed. After removing the running stitch I waited for two to four weeks before fitting the final glasses. This allows for tissue movement once the suture tension is removed.

The first transplant I did was during my residency. The patient was a young man with advanced keratoconus. He could not see any of the letters on the eye chart which meant that he was legally blind. He told me that he wanted to see better so that he could obtain a license to drive a car.

At that time, we kept corneal transplant patients in the hospital for three weeks with all but the last two days at strict bed rest. The attending surgeon who helped me with the case liked to use 10-O (very fine) twisted silk suture to sew in the graft. The surgery went well. Every day, for the next three weeks, we would check the eye, instill antibiotics drops and a drop to dilate the pupil and then put a fresh patch over the eye. Being in bed for three weeks often makes the patient weak, so the last two days in the hospital, the nurses were instructed to walk the patient in the hall. This was to enable him to walk to and from the car to get home after he left the hospital. A Hill Burton federal grant for care of indigent patients that was awarded to the Richmond Eye Hospital paid for his three weeks of hospitalization.

He did well after he left the hospital and in three months he was ready to have the sutures removed. Silk sutures make the wound heal faster, but they increase the chance of immune rejection. One month after I removed his sutures, he returned for me to order glasses for him.

Before I determined the needed power for his glasses, I checked his vision. He read all the way to the 20/20 line without any glasses. He had a perfect result. His operated eye saw perfectly without glasses.

I told him he could go back to work because he could see perfectly with his operated eye.

He asked, "What do you mean go back to work? I'm on total disability because I am legally blind!"

I told him that he was no longer totally blind so he could get a job and go to work. He stormed out of my office, yelling that I had ruined him, because he had been set for a life on total disability. I never saw him again. I do not know if he got a job or a driver's license, or if he managed to stay on welfare.

A perfect result from a corneal transplant is a rare event. Of the hundreds of transplants that I did, I can only remember three who did not need glasses of some sort to see well after their transplant.

The circular incision must heal exactly the same throughout the 360 degrees. If one stitch is too tight or too loose, or the wound heals unevenly, the cornea will be slightly warped and create astigmatism. In one study, the average astigmatism was 3.00 Diopters with a range from 1 to 6 Diopters. This amount of astigmatism almost always needs glasses. Although, I did have a young transplant patient with six Diopters of astigmatism at 90 degrees who read the same letters on the eye chart with, and without, glasses. Astigmatism at 90 degrees will compress the letters horizontally, but they may still be readable.

Since the cornea heals so slowly, the incision line stays fragile for many months after the operation. A patient of mine bumped his head on a car door getting out of a taxi. I had waited for sixteen months after the surgery to remove his sutures and the incident occurred six months after the sutures were removed. After he bumped his head, he felt something in his eye. He had split open the incision for about 90 degrees of the circle and one edge of his transplant had slipped forward. The incision line did not leak, but his eye felt rough. We had to re-suture the incision.

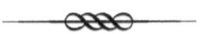

Another patient came back about six months after his surgery while he still had his sutures in place. The stitch broke and the lower half of the incision line ruptured. His eye was leaking, so I took him to the operating room and re-sutured the area that had ruptured. He told me the next day that he had been smoking pot and drinking all evening before he fell out of bed and hit his eye on the bedside table. I considered that extraordinary behavior that was outside of my usual instructions and precautions.

AGE-RELATED MACULAR DEGENERATION

One of the most frequent questions I get when I talk to people about eye problems is whether there is any new hope for patients with macular degeneration. The short answer is yes. The long answer is that there is a lot of research being done and some has promise. Some macular degeneration can be treated.

Age-related macular degeneration (ARMD or AMD) is the most common cause of permanent visual loss in people over the age of sixty. (Cataracts cause blindness that is very successfully treatable by surgery, so it is not permanent. Glaucoma causes blindness that often occurs before the age of sixty). ARMD is a degeneration of the retina that involves the center of the retina, the macula. It occurs in two types; "wet" and "dry" degeneration.

The dry type shows a collection of white spots within the retina in the macular area and develops irregular pigmentation as the retinal pigment layer, on the back of the retina, degenerates.

The rods and cones break down and vision is lost. The degenerated retina is filled with irregular clumps of pigment. About 85% of ARMD is of the dry type. There is presently no successful treatment of the dry type of ARMD once it has occurred. There are treatments to avoid or postpone ARMD.

In the wet type, new vessels beneath the retina leak serum into the retina and it swells or the retina detaches locally. This also causes the retinal pigment layer to degenerate and scatter pigment.

There are hemorrhages in and beneath the retina. The basement membrane of the retina shows breaks that facilitate fluid leakage into the retina. This form of degeneration may respond to simple laser treatment to burn areas of leakage, but this treatment is rarely done now.

I believe that ARMD has a vascular cause and that is why it only involves the macular region. The retina has two blood supplies; the choroid from behind, and the retinal vessels on the front surface. The rods and cones are more tightly packed in the macula, especially the cones of the fovea, the center of the macula.

This gives us the sharpest vision in these areas, but also requires more nutrition and oxygen.

The retinal vessels do not extend to the foveal area so there is no blood supply for oxygen and nutrients to the front of the fovea. The fovea receives oxygen and nutrients from the choroidal vasculature behind it. The peripheral retina has the two blood supplies—retinal vessels and choroidal vessels. Disease of the choroidal vessels will affect the macula more than the peripheral retina.

Tissue around blocked vessels makes a substance, VEGF (vascular endothelial growth factor), that causes new vessels to grow in that area. These new vessels are thin walled and leaky so the surrounding area collects fluid, making it "wet."

The point that I always emphasize to patients with ARMD is that the disease only involves the macula area. The remainder of the retina is not involved, so peripheral vision remains intact.

Unfortunately, peripheral vision is not as sharp as central vision.

A patient with advanced ARMD can walk through a room full of furniture without running into anything. They can get around just fine, but they cannot read and have difficulty watching television.

They cannot drive because their vision straight ahead is blurred or blocked in the area where the driver sees the road.

Recognition of age-related macular degeneration

How do I know if I have macular degeneration? Noticeable symptoms of macular degeneration begin as small areas of visual distortion that are not noticeable to the patient unless they are looking at something that has a fine, but regular pattern that is distorted by the change in the macula. As the areas become larger, print is harder to read because some areas are indistinct. As these areas of degeneration become larger and more numerous, print must be larger to be read. Eventually the bad spots may blot out whole words or areas of text on a page.

People's faces become blurred to the point of non recognition.

The face is blurred, but the ears look OK. The center of the television is all blurred, but the TV is still there. Looking at a cup on the table may make it disappear. Looking to the side of the cup, the person can see the cup in their side vision.

I tell patients to get low vision magnifiers when they first start to have trouble. Some of these can be purchased at drug stores, optical shops or through the local blind assistance office or through catalog sales. Ophthalmologists can advise about which ones will work best for the patient and order them for the patient.

There is an industry around low vision aids. It runs from magnifying lenses and telescopic lenses to check book masks, large button telephones, and television magnified reading devices. Computers can be used to read text with voice simulators.

There are some common sense remedies that help to adapt to this loss of central vision. I told my patients that, when they want to see a face, look over the person's shoulder. This puts the face in the intact peripheral vision. They should put a big plant next to the TV set and look at it when they watch TV. They will not see the plant, but they will see the screen in their side vision so they can follow along. They will not be able to read the commercials or graphics on the news, but they can follow soap operas and sit coms just fine. Of course, I have always maintained that one can follow soap operas without seeing the screen at all.

There is a miniature telescope that is under investigation at Massachusetts Eye and Ear Infirmary and several other teaching centers. It is implanted within the eye. It enlarges everything, which makes the effective blind spot smaller. Early results with this implantable telescope are encouraging. The FDA has approved this device for implantation by the physicians who performed the first studies at several centers. If this produces good results, the number of surgeons who can implant this device will probably be expanded.

Some states allow the use of telescopic glasses for driving a car. These telescopes magnify the central area and make it easier to see, but the enlarged area covers some of the peripheral area.

A child running into the street or a car approaching from the side might be obscured by this enlarged area. I do not recommend using telescopic lenses for driving. Telescopes of various designs help reading, viewing television, and looking up telephone numbers.

When I first saw a patient with multiple drussen, the little white spots, I gave them a card with a grid of white lines on a black background, called an Amsler Grid. These lines are straight and cross perpendicular to each other. There is a dot in the center of the grid.

The patient tests one eye at a time covering the other with the palm of their hand, not their fingers. (Peeking through the fingers may improve the vision in the covered eye.) They look at the center dot and see if any of the lines on the card are distorted or missing. Wavy, blurred, or missing lines indicate an area of disease in the retina.

The patient can mark areas of the grid with a pencil where lines are wavy or missing. As they look at the card every week, they can see if these areas are changing. Changes indicate activity in the disease that may need treatment, or at least mean a return visit to the ophthalmologist to see if treatment is needed. I recommend that the patient place the Amsler Grid on the inside of the medicine cabinet door so that every time they brush their teeth, they can quickly check for changes in the patterns.

Many remedies have been tried to prevent, or slow, the progress of macular degeneration. They include taking fish oils, aspirin, steroids, non-steroidal anti-inflammatories such as Advil, and using orange colored glasses. The orange colored (blue free) glasses help to sharpen the image by removing blue light, but the other things just mentioned do not seem to help. Shooters often wear yellow or orange glasses to sharpen the target and reduce glare from the sights. Yellow or orange glasses are often advertised on late night television and in catalogs. They actually improve vision in early ARMD.

Prevention of age-related macular degeneration

At this time there is no effective medical or surgical treatment for dry ARMD that will improve vision or arrest visual loss. The best thing available is to try to prevent it. Risk factors such as high blood pressure and smoking should be dealt with. People with hypertension are one and a half times more likely to get ARMD.

Smoking doubles the risk.

Taking a mixture of vitamins and selected minerals has been shown in a large, nationwide study to slow the progression of macular degeneration in many patients. This study, called the ARED Study for Age Related Eye Disease Study, was organized and conducted by the National Eye Institute. The ARED formula of vitamins and minerals plus Lutein is available, over the counter, at drugstores. Some brand names include: Ocuvites, Eye Vites, AMD Vitamins, PreserVision, VisiVite, and ARMD Complete Eye Vitamins. There are many generics, some of which have added other drugs that have not been proven to help.

Many doctors think that a healthy diet with fruits and vegetables that furnish free radical scavengers and vitamins may help. These foods are rich in the vitamins and minerals in the ARED formula.

> I do not yet have macular degeneration and I do not smoke or have high blood pressure, but I take Centrum Silver for Senior Men every day. It has almost everything that is in the ARED formula plus other vitamins that are good for general health and it costs less.

Treatment of age-related macular degeneration

Once you have wet ARMD, especially if it is progressing, there are modern treatments that have shown promise in stopping or retarding the progression of macular degeneration. About 15% of ARMD patients have the wet type. Recent studies have shown that early treatment is more effective in arresting the progression of wet ARMD. The treatments fall into three categories; 1) direct laser photocoagulation, 2) photo dynamic therapy (PDT), and 3) anti-neovascular treatment.

Direct laser photocoagulation involves locating a neovascular membrane, between the retina and the choroid, by Fluorescein angiography; then burning it with the laser to photocoagulate the tissue and vessels to stop the leakage from the vessels. This causes damage to the retina and is rarely used because better treatments have been developed.

Photo dynamic therapy is done by injecting a drug called Visudyne into the blood stream and allowing it to circulate to the eye. Visudyne is attracted to the retinal and choroidal pigment, enhancing the effect of laser treatment. A broad beam laser is directed to the macular area where it activates the Visudyne.

The activated Visudyne then destroys the new vessels, stopping the leak and drying the macula. Somewhere between 40% and 60%

of wet ARMD patients have neovascularization that can be treated with this method.

The third type of treatment is directed at destroying or preventing recurrence of the neovascularization. Damaged vessels in the retina produce Vascular Endothelial Growth Factor (VEGF, pronounced veg-F) that encourages new vessel growth.

By using anti-VEGF drugs the vessels are inhibited. There are four drugs on the market today that are used to fight VEGF. They are Lucentis (runibizumab), Avastin (bevacizumab, Macugen (pegaptanib), and Eylea (aflibercept). Recently, Avastin has been removed from the market for treating ARMD, but it is still available to treat cancer. Some outside pharmacies may still be making up the ocular dosage. A recent study showed that Eylea may improve the results obtained from several injections of Lucentis.

The four medications vary slightly in complication rates, side effects, cost, and dosage. They can improve vision slightly in about one third of cases and stabilize up to 95% of the eyes treated. The eyes that continue to deteriorate do so at a slower rate.

These drugs are injected directly into the eye. This scares many patients, but the needle is small and the eye is anesthetized so most people do not feel the injection. The injection must be repeated every month to be effective. The makers of Eylea claim that the injection rate can be reduced to every two months after the first three monthly injections. Anti-VEGF therapy works only in wet, age-related macular degeneration.

Some retina specialists use both photo dynamic therapy and anti-VEGF treatments to control wet ARMD.

Remember, ARMD does not cause complete blindness; the peripheral vision remains. Healthy life style and good diet or special vitamins can prevent or decrease visual loss. There are treatments available if you have the wet type of ARMD. At the first sign of ARMD, you should see a retina specialist and take their advice.

Central areolar choroidal sclerosis

A disease that is often confused with age-related macular degeneration is central areolar choroidal sclerosis. This starts as circles of degeneration in the macular region. These circles are not limited to the macular region and eventually may involve the entire retina leading to total blindness.

Central areolar choroidal sclerosis is transmitted by either dominant or recessive means. This disease manifests in middle age with progressive visual loss. Atrophy of the retinal pigment layer may be extensive before the vision loss is apparent.

UVEITIS

Uveitis is the term for inflammation of any part of the uveal tract. The uveal tract includes the iris, the ciliary body, and the choroid. These are all pigmented parts of the eye that make up the middle layer of the posterior eye and extend anteriorly to form the ciliary body and iris.

The iris is a flat circle of tissue which contains a hole in the center called the pupil. It contains several layers of tissue with lacy stroma anteriorly and a pigment layer posteriorly. The stroma contains vessels and both radial and circumferential muscle fibers.

These muscles dilate and constrict the pupil. The amount of pigment in the iris determines the color of the iris. Blonds usually have blue eyes; brunettes usually have brown eyes; and albino people have grey or pink eyes. In Pittsburgh, there is a belief that blue-eyed; dark haired girls are descendents of Italian and Irish marriages.

Chronic inflammation in an eye can cause the iris to darken.

Both irises (iridies) are usually the same color. Several conditions may cause one iris to be different from the other, i.e., one blue and the other brown. This is called heterochromia iridis. This term can also be used to describe the condition where one part of the iris is lighter or darker than another part in the same eye.

Congenital Horner's syndrome involving impaired sympathetic innervation of the iris makes the involved iris lighter, either blue or grey. Acquired Horner's syndrome from injury or a tumor in the neck does not have heterochromia. A melanoma within the eye causes the iris in that eye to turn darker. Sometimes one iris is darker than the other with no pathological reason. Both Julius Caesar and George Washington are said to have had heterochromia of the iris. Some patients with a chronic iritis will develop heterochromia.

Iritis (inflammation of the iris) causes the white of the eye to become pink to red in appearance. This redness is concentrated at the edge of the cornea and is called ciliary flush. The pupil may be slightly dilated or constricted. The iris vessels become dilated and leak protein and white blood cells into the anterior chamber of the eye. These show up in the slit lamp beam as flare and cells.

Flare is a haze, like headlights through fog that is seen in the beam of the slit lamp. Cells are seen in the slit lamp beam as dust floating in the sunlight or snow flurries in the headlight beams.

They drift in the aqueous humor in the eye.

The main symptom of iritis is photophobia (pain from bright light). The patient may be very uncomfortable in room light or sun light. Vision may be dim or blurred.

Iritis and uveitis occur in two forms which are differentiated by the presence or absence of clumps of cells called granulomas, so there is granulomatous iritis and non-granulomatous iritis.

Granulomatous uveitis

There are many causes of granulomatous uveitis. The most common forms of granulomatous uveitis are from tuberculosis, toxoplasmosis, and Sarcoidosis. These usually involve all parts of the uveal tract. The granulomatous nature of these is manifested by the appearance of white spots on the posterior surface of the cornea.

The spots are found on the lower half of the cornea with the highest point at the center of the cornea. The convection currents in the anterior chamber flow up in front the warm iris and then down behind the cooler cornea. When the downward flow hits the cornea as it recedes toward the limbus in the lower half, the clumps of white blood cells collide with the cornea and stick to it.

These diseases may cause white spots to form on the iris and lens. The inflammation may cause the iris to adhere to the lens.

When the pupil dilates, it is stuck to the lens in places so that the pupil dilates unevenly and the pupil is not round. When the uveitis persists, the pupil may be stuck permanently to the lens causing a small pupil. If these adhesions are broken, using strong dilating drops to pull the iris loose, a ring of pigment may be left, adhering to the lens. This ring is called a Vosious' Ring.

Adhesion of the iris to the lens may cause glaucoma by blocking the egress of fluid from the posterior chamber through the pupil. This pushes the iris forward, blocking the angle and raising the pressure.

Regardless of the exact cause, the reaction is similar. To determine the cause of the uveitis, it is necessary to perform a battery of laboratory testing. Since several of the diseases that can cause granulomatous uveitis can be life threatening, it is important to do a complete evaluation so that serious diseases can be treated.

Chest X-rays can diagnose tuberculosis and sarcoidosis. Skin testing must be done for TB because TB can exist in other organs outside the lungs such as the spine and the kidneys. Immune titers can be done for many infectious disorders and autoimmune diseases.

History, or concurrent manifestations, of infectious diseases from bacteria, viruses, fungi, and parasites may indicate the causative agent. These include herpes, Rubella, Lime disease, Cryptococcus, or Toxocara. Some of these diseases can, and should, be treated.

Treatment for granulomatous uveitis is usually directed systemically at the causative agent. Ocular treatment is directed toward reduction of complications. To prevent the iris from sticking to the lens, the pupil is dilated. This also reduces the pain from iris muscle spasm brought on by the inflammation. Topical eye drops and subconjunctival injections of steroids help in uveitis caused by non infectious causes, but must be used sparingly, if at all, in tuberculosis and fungal diseases. Acute viral diseases must run their courses, but systemic anti virals such as acyclovir can be used against chronic viral diseases such as herpes.

Non-granulomatous uveitis

The major cause of non-granulomatous uveitis is autoimmune diseases such as rheumatoid arthritis, ankylosing spondylitis, ulcerative colitis, Chron's disease, and psoriasis. Leukemia and lymphoma may also manifest initially as uveitis.

Many people have their first episode of non-granulomatous uveitis before they are forty years old. An extensive workup does not reveal the cause and the uveitis goes away after several weeks and does not recur. Because of this, many doctors do not work up the first episode of non-granulomatous uveitis. If the uveitis recurs, they do the work up.

Since the most common cause is rheumatoid disease, we check for certain serum antibodies, particularly HLA-B27. HLA antibodies are used to tissue type patients for tissue matching before transplants, but certain antibodies are known to be common in specific diseases. The rheumatoid factor and other rheumatoid indicators are also checked.

Another form of non granulomatous uveitis is from intraocular foreign bodies. Iron will rust and cause inflammation and damage the retina. Copper and brass will damage the retina and turn the iris blue-green. Retained vegetable matter from puncture wounds will cause chronic inflammation.

> I had a sixty-plus-year-old patient who came to me because he had cataracts. After I removed the first cataract, he did well for several weeks. At about the third week, he began having cells floating in his anterior chamber. I thought

he might have a delayed infection caused by mild acting bacteria.

I gave him the medication to treat the infection, but he became worse. His vision deteriorated and his retina began showing hemorrhages and infiltrates that looked like herpes simplex in an AIDS patient, but he did not have AIDS.

We sent him to a major university to check the cells in his eye for autoimmune markers for a tumor. He was found to have markers on the cells for a lymphoma in his brain. At that time, an MRI scan of the brain did not show a tumor. Three weeks later he was admitted to the hospital because of a seizure. A repeat MRI scan showed three areas of brain lymphoma. Two weeks later he was dead from multiple brain tumors. This presentation of a tumor as uveitis is called Masquerade syndrome and occurs with several different tumors.

Sympathetic ophthalmia

There is a specific type of posterior uveitis that happens after a significant injury to the eye, usually involving the iris or choroid within the eye. Several weeks after repair of the eye, the vision becomes blurred in both eyes. There is pain on movement of the eyes and they are tender to touch. This uveitis involves the choroid and the retina. It I called sympathetic ophthalmia. If it is not treated the eye can become blind. It is caused by an autoimmune response to the injured choroidal tissue. The antibodies try to destroy the choroid as a foreign substance.

Since birth, the uvea has been isolated from the body by the blood-brain, or blood-eye, barrier, so the immune system does not know it is there. The trauma exposed the uvea to the immune system that did not recognize the uvea as "self" and therefore, set out to destroy it. Unfortunately, the immune system cannot tell the uveal tissue in the uninjured eye from that in the injured eye so both eyes are attacked.

Treatment of sympathetic ophthalmia is suppression by steroids; topical, local injection, and systemic by pills in relatively high doses. There is new evidence that some anticancer drugs may be effective.

When an eye is severely injured and there is little, or no, hope for restoring vision, most ophthalmologists will remove the injured eye before the immune response has had a chance to happen, which is within the first seven to ten days after the injury. I usually repaired the eye to determine if vision could be restored.

If the eye could not see light on the day after surgery, I told the patient that it was best to remove the eye immediately, rather than risk a reaction in the other eye.

This approach had two benefits. First, sometimes useful vision was restored. Second, the patient had the opportunity to see that vision had not been restored before deciding to remove the eye and sometimes a few days to think about the consequences.

> My father lost his left eye and left thumb in a hunting accident when he was seventeen. He was still able to practice general surgery for thirty years with only one eye. I have always been amazed by how well people can function with just one eye, because they should lose all depth perception.

Once the immune reaction has occurred, if there is useful vision in the injured eye, the injured eye is not removed. It may have the best vision of the two eyes once the immune response has run its course.

Posterior scleritis

Another autoimmune response in the eye involves the sclera.

Posterior scleritis is most common in patients with rheumatoid diseases. Rheumatoid disease also causes an anterior scleritis that thins the sclera in round spots, allowing the uvea to show through as a dark blue or black spot on the sclera. The sclera may become so thin that it perforates with the escape of ocular contents. It is called necrotizing scleromalacia.

> A patient came to me in Texas with the complaint that she had a dull boring pain behind both of her eyes. It was present all of the time and kept her awake at night. When she looked to the side, the pain was worse. When I examined her, the eye appeared completely normal. There was no reaction in the retina or choroid to explain the pain.
>
> I conducted an ultrasound examination of the eye and found that her posterior sclera was almost twice a thick a normal in both eyes. This told me that she had a posterior scleritis. This as almost always linked to a rheumatoid disease.
>
> Oral steroids controlled the pain in several days and the dosage was slowly tapered to the minimum dose that would control her symptoms.

ACQUIRED (ADULT) STRABISMUS OR MUSCLE PALSY

There are a number of causes of gradual or sudden muscle paralysis of the extraocular muscles. They manifest as misalignment of the eyes and double vision.

The six muscles that move each eye are the four rectus muscles that move each eye up, down, left, and right, and the two oblique muscles of each eye. The superior oblique muscle rotates the eye around the anterior-posterior axis of the eye to pull the top of the eye toward the nose and moves the front of the eye away from the nose. The inferior oblique muscle rotates the eye around the anterior-posterior axis of the eye to move the top of the eye away from the nose and it also moves the front of the eye away from the nose.

Since these palsies occur in adults, after the age when the brain can learn to suppress the image from one eye, these patients see double.

In palsy of the third cranial nerve, the paralyzed eye will turn down and out. The third nerve supplies three rectus muscles, medial, superior and inferior, and the inferior oblique muscle.

They all become lax. The lateral rectus and the superior oblique are still active, pulling the involved eye down and out. This causes double vision, if both eyes are open. The images will be crossed (the image seen on the right is the one seen by the left eye.) and it is vertically displaced upward because the left eye was down. If the separation is very far apart, the brain may not recognize the widely displaced image, so there is no sensation of double vision.

Since the third nerve also enervates the levator palpebrae, the muscle that raises the upper eyelid, the eyelid will not open, so the patient does not see double until the eyelid is raised.

The most common causes of third nerve palsy are diabetes, cerebral aneurysms, hypertension and trauma. Diabetes and hypertension are vascular diseases that affect the blood supply.

Aneurysms and trauma involve pressure on the nerve, somewhere between where it emerges from the brainstem and the path through the orbit. Since the vessels are within the nerve and the nerve fibers to the pupil run in a bundle on the surface of the nerve, hypertension and diabetes rarely involve the pupillary fibers.

Aneurysms from the circle of Willis, the ring of blood vessels around the base of the brain, often push against the third nerve as it passes beneath the brain. Trauma to the head may make the brain shift and smash the third nerve. The history of trauma or lack thereof, helps differentiate between aneurysms and trauma.

To differentiate between an aneurysm and diabetes requires testing the pupil responses to light or simply observing pupil size.

If the pupil is normal, the injury is probably vascular—vascular occlusive diseases like diabetes or hypertension. If the pupil is dilated, there is pressure on the outside of the nerve, either from an aneurysm or from trauma. The aneurysm is a neurosurgical emergency to be seen by a neurologist or neurosurgeon the same day. A pupil sparing third nerve begs for a medical work up for diabetes and/or hypertension or other vascular diseases within a week from the onset.

Rare causes of third nerve palsies include meningioma and cavernous sinus disease.

When a person experiences vertical double vision or vision in which one image seems to be rotated with respect to the other, the most likely cause is a fourth cranial nerve (CN IV) palsy. The most common causes are trauma and vascular. The forth nerve is very susceptible to trauma, especially frontal blows to the head which throw the brain forward within the cranium. This happens during injuries like going over the handle bars of a bicycle after a sudden stop and landing on the forehead, or running into a wall.

Unexplained forth nerve palsy in a child should prompt consideration of cerebellar tumors.

Examination of a person with a fourth cranial nerve, (CN IV) palsy shows the eye higher on the involved side than on the other.

The superior oblique or trochlear muscle rotates the top of the eye toward the nose and pushes it down. When it is paralyzed, the inferior oblique is unopposed, so it pushes the front of the eye up. The rotation of the inferior oblique is also unopposed so the eye rotates and images from the two eyes do not line up. Once the vertical alignment of the eye is disrupted, any latent horizontal misalignment tendency may cause the eyes to cross or deviate outward, complicating the diagnosis.

Damage to the sixth cranial nerve (CN VI) is the most common of the ocular nerve palsies. It is the longest of the cranial nerves to the eye and has more ways it can be injured. The palsy can occur in one or both eyes. The eyes may be crossed and cannot move outward past straight ahead when trying to look to the same side as the eye (right eye looking right). The major causes include trauma, diabetes, increased intracranial pressure, brain tumors, vascular disease, and meningitis.

The occurrence of bilateral sixth nerve palsy and swelling of the optic nerve (papilledema) in the absence of any other neurological sign is an indication of increased intracranial pressure from pseudotumor cerebrii. Treatments include removal of drug related causes, draining cerebral spinal fluid by lumbar puncture, diuretics to inhibit fluid production, and even surgery in the eye socket or a cerebral shunt to drain the fluid.

A number of special ocular syndromes such as Duane's syndrome and myasthenia gravis may mimic bilateral sixth nerve palsies.

Myasthenia gravis often presents as eye muscle weakness which is intermittent. A patient with alternating ptosis, a drooping eyelid that is present one day in the right eye and the next day in the left eye is almost certainly myasthenia. An episode of double vision from a single muscle or one that gets worse when the person is tired may be myasthenia. Having the person look up for a long time will test for myasthenia because the lid will begin to sag after a few seconds. Repeating the test again and again will shorten the time before the lid drops. A definite diagnosis can be made by doing the Tensilon (edruphonium) test. In myasthenia, the acetylcholine neurotransmitter is metabolized too rapidly.

Tensilon blocks the acetylcholine esterase that destroys the acetylcholine, allowing the muscle to contract better. If the patient has myasthenia gravis, the eye movement problem will improve with Tensilon.

The treatment of ocular nerve palsies depends on the underlying disease. Traumatic nerve injuries often regenerate. The injured nerve grows out through the sheaths of the dead nerves at a rate of about one centimeter per month. This translates to six to twelve months in most cases. Since the paralysis will go away when the nerve regenerates, surgery to move the eyes is not indicated.

Diplopia (seeing double) is very disturbing, especially when reading. I advise patients to cover one eye and read all they want.

One way to do this is to cover the spectacle lens for one eye with several layers of cellophane tape. This blurs the vision to block that eye, but it is not apparent to the casual observer. Some patients prefer to wear a patch, available at drug stores, to look like a pirate. Another solution is to pull a facial tissue behind the lens on one side of spectacles so that it blocks the vision from that eye. When you have finished reading, remove the tissue, blow your nose and throw it away. When the nerve regeneration reaches the muscle, the separation of the images becomes less and may resolve completely.

Another treatment is to use prisms that press on to the back of the person's glasses. If the paralysis is partial, this may help the person to fuse the images from the two eyes, however, people tend to need more and more prism, with time, to overcome the double vision and eventually need more than can be provided with press on prisms.

If the paralysis in permanent, as when nerves are cut and not rejoined, ocular muscle surgery may be considered to realign the eyes. When one muscle is paralyzed and the opposing muscle is not, the unopposed active muscle tension will stretch the paralyzed muscle and pull the eye out of alignment so the surgery may have to be repeated.

One other problem that causes acquired, traumatic, double vision is the blowout fracture. If a fist, racket ball, baseball, or similar object, hits the front of the eye, it occludes the front opening of the eye socket and then increases the pressure in the eye socket. This pressure may fracture the bones of the eye socket and push the contents of the eye socket through the fracture line.

When the pressure is released, the socket contents may try to return to the socket, but get trapped in the fracture. The most common walls to blow out are the floor and the nasal wall of the socket. Entrapment of tissue is common in floor fractures. If the muscle or the ligaments that run through the orbit are caught in the wound, they restrict the inferior rectus muscle and the eye is unable to look up or may be trapped in down gaze. This causes vertical double vision.

The correction of this usually requires surgery to release the trapped tissues and restore the floor of the socket. An incision is made through the lower eyelid to approach the lower rim of the eye socket. The periosteum covering the bone of the floor is elevated from the bone and the tissue is pulled through the fracture, if possible. Sheet silicone or other materials may be used to cover the fracture so the muscle does not return to the fracture and the eyeball cannot sink within the socket if part of the floor is absent or depressed. Double vision may persist for weeks or months after this surgical repair due to injury to the muscle.

Most surgeons will not operate on a blow out fracture if there is no double vision or the double vision is only in up gaze. The chance of creating double vision by doing the surgery outweighs the benefits of fixing the fracture.

DIABETES AND THE EYE

Diabetes Mellitus is a disease which affects many organs and tissues in the body. It does this mainly by changes in the blood vessels. Dr. Phillip Poffenbarger, at University of Texas Medical Branch (UTMB) in Galveston, explained it to my residents years ago when I was at Utmb in Texas. According to him, the body is constantly replacing old membranes in vessels and organs for all parts of the body. These membranes are composed of proteins that are broken down by enzymes and removed.

They are then replaced by new proteins that link together to form new membranes. This is much like chipping an asphalt road, recycling the asphalt, and laying it down as new pavement.

Normally these membranes do not contain sugars, but when the blood sugar is high, as it is in diabetes, the sugar molecules may be improperly incorporated into the membranes. The enzymes that break the protein bonds in the first stage of replacing the membranes cannot break the bonds between proteins and sugars, halting the process, so part of the membrane is not removed. The new membrane is laid down over the remnants that could not be broken down, so the membrane becomes thick.

Most organs and blood vessels are made of cells attached to membranes. The nutrients and metabolites pass through these thin membranes to nourish and cleanse the organs. When the membranes become thickened because there are protein to sugar remnants, the membranes do not work properly and the function of the organ or blood vessel is impaired.

The organs most affected by diabetes are the heart, kidneys, and nervous system, including the eyes.

Diabetes can cause paralysis of the ocular muscles by damage to the nerves that control the eye movements. Nerves contain tiny capillaries that carry blood through the nerves. When these vessels develop micro aneurysms or become occluded, the nerve is damaged and the impulses cannot travel along the nerve.

The most common extra ocular nerve involved in diabetes is the third cranial nerve. It controls the superior, inferior, and medial rectus muscles and the inferior oblique muscle that move the eye up, down, toward the nose, and up and outward, looking away from the nose respectively. It also controls the muscle that opens the eye, the levator muscle in the upper eyelid. When diabetes blocks this nerve, the eyelid is closed and the eyeball is rotated down and out toward the temple.

In third cranial nerve palsy caused by diabetes, the pupil usually remains reactive to light. The fibers that control the pupil are in a band on the outside of the nerve. Since the nerve is also nourished by the cerebral spinal fluid, the pupil fibers are usually spared. When an aneurysm is crushing the third nerve, it will usually block the fibers that control the pupil, making the pupil unresponsive to light. (The pupil will not constrict when light is shown in to the eye.)

Diabetic infarction (vessel closure) to the fourth and sixth cranial nerves will cause palsy of the superior oblique muscle and the lateral rectus muscles respectively.

Palsy of the superior oblique muscle causes the eye to turn up and out away from the nose while a lateral rectus muscle palsy keeps the eye from turning out toward the temple.

Within the eye, there are early signs of diabetes. Small breaks in blood vessels cause small hemorrhages. These are usually deep in the retina so they appear round. The vessels may stretch to form aneurysms. These are also red spots on the retina. Hemorrhages are not confined so the edges are fuzzy. Aneurysms are confined so the spots have sharp edges as a round red spot. Areas of the retina near a blocked capillary are oxygen starved so they appear as a white fuzzy spot called a cotton wool spot.

Diabetes plays a role in the infarctions of the central retina artery and vein. These cause immediate loss of vision within a few minutes. A central retinal artery blockage will cause permanent loss of vision within ten to twenty minutes if the artery is not reopened. Blockage of the oxygen supply to the retina kills the retina tissue.

In retinal vein occlusion, the blood flow is greatly diminished, but vision may be restored gradually after the vein opens again.

People with central retinal vein occlusion may develop new vessels on the retina several weeks to months after the occlusion.

These need to be treated by an ophthalmologist with either the laser or the new anti-VEGF medications used in Age Related Macular Degeneration, ARMD. Diabetes affects the capillaries of the retina. The capillaries in the retina form a reticular pattern which permeates the retina to supply oxygen containing blood. When these vessels become blocked by the changes of diabetes, parts of the retina have a decreased blood and oxygen supply. This causes the retina to produce a chemical called Vascular Endothelial Growth Factor (VEGF). This chemical causes new vessels to grow into the area to correct the lack of blood and oxygen supplied to that part of the retina. These vessels grow on the surface of the retina, between the surface of the retina and the vitreous rather than within the retina where the normal vessels would be. Because of this position, these vessels often break causing small hemorrhages. They also leak fluid from the blood stream that collects in the retina as edema fluid. This often occurs in the central macular area, interfering with vision straight ahead.

The new vessels that grow on the surface of the retina occur in patches where the blood supply has been compromised and also around the optic nerve. They are called NVD (neovascularization of the disk), when the new vessels are around the optic nerve or disk. If they occur anywhere else on the retina, they are called NVE or neovascularization elsewhere.

The patient cannot tell when they have new vessels on the surface of the retina unless they cause a large hemorrhage. People with diabetes should be checked by an ophthalmologist at least once a year to see if they have new vessel formation. Once new vessels are seen, the visits must be more frequent to determine when treatment is necessary.

If the eye is forming new vessels, diabetic retinopathy, this process can be stopped by laser treatments. The goal of the laser treatments is to destroy the areas of the retina that produce the vasoproliferative substance, VEGF, by burning the retina with a laser.

To find these avascular areas, sterile fluorescein solution is injected into a vein on the arm. The fluorescein is carried in the blood to the eye where it fills the retinal vessels. Fluorescein gives off an apple green light when it is excited by cobalt blue light.

The vascular tree glows green when it is full of excited fluorescein.

By photographing the retina in black and white, we can get a good picture of the tiny capillaries of the retina and find black areas were the capillaries are blocked. The fluorescein is removed from the blood by the kidneys and eliminated in the urine. Many patients have been surprised when their urine glowed green in the ultraviolet lights used to sanitize public restrooms. Without the ultraviolet light, the fluorescein is a brownish yellow.

Hundreds of small burns are made in the retina, concentrating on the avascular areas. Once this tissue is dead, VEGF is not produced and the vessels will shrink and go away, decreasing the chance of hemorrhage into the eye.

Each burn kills a small portion of retina and makes a tiny blind spot. Most people who have had laser photocoagulation of the retina do not notice these blind spots. The brain fills in the gaps and if both eyes are seeing, the image from one eye fills in the gaps from the other eye.

If these vessels have been allowed to grow, they may cause a major hemorrhage into the vitreous body. These hemorrhages may organize into a membrane that is opaque, usually white or yellow in color. These membranes can block almost all vision to the extent that the person sees only whether a light that is shown into the eye is on or off. Before about 1970, there was no effective treatment for these organized membranes in the vitreous. With the advent of vitrectomy, it was possible to place a tiny instrument into the eye to nibble these membranes and remove them from the eye without damaging the retina.

In the mid to late seventies, I removed many membranes from the eyes of diabetics who had been blind for as long as twenty years. Many of these people still had useful vision once the membranes were removed. Some could even read books or newspapers.

One patient told me that he had seen his three-year-old granddaughter for the first time. The little girl's mother had been about three years old when he last saw her.

In some of the patients, the diabetes had destroyed most of their retina, so removing the membranes by vitrectomy did not restore their vision. However, most patients benefitted from having these membranes removed. Many were able to move about independently and return to work. Most were able to watch television and read again.

Patients with diabetes may develop cholesterol deposits in the retina. Serum leaks from diabetic vessels into the retina. The cholesterol remains in the retina when the fluid is reabsorbed.

> I had a patient with advanced diabetic retinopathy and a cholesterol level around five hundred mg/dl, (Normal 125-200 mg/dl). Most of his retina was covered with yellow cholesterol deposits. His diabetic retinopathy could not be treated with the laser because of the cholesterol plaques. His vision was reduced to 20/400 in both eyes. He died of a heart attack shortly after I saw him.

New vessel formation in diabetes may also affect the iris. Tiny vessels grow on the surface of the iris near the opening for the pupil. A membrane forms between the vessels. Contraction of that membrane may cause the edges of the pupil to curl. If the eye is operated for cataract while these vessels are present, the vessels break and hemorrhage during the surgery. The bleeding blocks the surgeon's view and makes the surgery very difficult, if not impossible.

These iris vessels usually disappear weeks after the retina is adequately treated with photocoagulation. I watched one cataract operation in which the vessels in the iris were not noticed before the surgery. As soon as the eye was opened, the vessels began to ooze blood. The surgery, that was supposed to take twenty to thirty minutes, lasted for over two hours, as the surgeon fought the bleeding. This was a demonstration case at an ocular surgery meeting and proved very embarrassing to the course director.

The incidence of glaucoma is greater in patients with diabetes that in the normal population. This is mostly the open angle type of glaucoma.

Dr. Naseem Ansari, a Ph.D. candidate in my department in Texas, demonstrated that cataract formation in diabetic rats could be delayed by 100% of the normal time (twice the usual time) by feeding them a diet high in free radical scavengers such as vitamin C and BHT, a preservative in snack foods.

People with diabetes have been known to form dense cataracts, almost overnight. Diabetic patients are known to have a high osmolarity, (concentration of ions) in the fluid in the eye.

The classic theory is that this high osmolarity causes the lens to become a cataract. Another theory is that there is also a high concentration of free radicals in the eye that cause the formation of the cataract. Dr. Ansari's work points to the latter, although the commonly believed dogma is that diabetic cataract formation is related to osmolarity.

The need for frequent eye exams in people with diabetes is so great that most insurance policies and Medicare will allow one free eye exam per year for anyone with diabetes.

I have seen many patients, who do not know that they have diabetes, who have come to see me because they cannot read with their bifocals and they have blurred vision at distance. They are usually between forty and sixty years old and have noticed a rather sudden change in vision.

Upon examination, they are found to have a shift of one to three Diopters in the farsighted direction in the glasses they need. Dr. Cam Sternberg told me about this change and said that he always sent these patients for a glucose tolerance test to see if they had adult onset diabetes. Almost all of these patients had diabetes.

They were started on treatment and soon returned to their original measurement for glasses. This took about six weeks in most patients, about the same amount of time that it takes hemoglobin A1C to return to normal after the control of diabetes is achieved. (Hemoglobin A1C is produced when blood sugar is high, so it is tested to determine if there are spikes in the blood sugar level between the normal readings reported by the patient.)

Classic teaching in ophthalmology is that diabetic acidosis causes myopia. This comes from a patient with near diabetic coma blood sugar levels, described by Sir Stewart Duke-Elder in his classic System of Ophthalmology. That person was found to become myopic.

The optometric literature is full of reports of diabetic animals and people who have a hyperopic shift, but attempts to report these patients in ophthalmology literature were refused on the basis of the "common knowledge" that diabetes causes myopia.

> Our contact lens optician came into my administrative office one morning and told me that he had suddenly developed blurred vision. He had checked himself and found out that he had a two Diopter shift in his glasses

toward farsightedness. I told him about Dr. Sternberg and some of my patients and suggested that he get checked for diabetes. The next week he came to me to tell me that he was found to be a Type II diabetic and had been started on oral hypoglycemic medication. Six weeks later he was back in his old glasses. He went on a strict diet and lost about thirty pounds and was able to stop his diabetic medications.

His glasses remained the same until he went off of his diet and regained the thirty pounds and had to return to his diabetic medications.

Obesity seems to play major role in the onset of type II diabetes. Many studies have demonstrated that diabetes can be controlled by diet and exercise. However, the same studies showed that most patients do not have the self control to continue the diet and exercise regimen after the study is over, so they soon return to poorly controlled diabetes.

THYROID EYE DISEASE

Patients with hyperthyroid disease can have many eye problems. Some patients have eye signs and symptoms without demonstrable systemic disease. These patients are said to have Grave's Eye Disease. The cause of hyperthyroid disease is thought to be autoimmune. The endocrinology is very complex.

Some patients with hyperthyroid disease have only minor irritation and dry eyes while others have prominent eyes, strange eyelid movements, double vision, corneal ulcers, blindness, and the inability to move the eyes in unison,. One of my classmates in medical school used to try to make everyone nervous before an exam by saying he could not remember all of the twenty-seven eye signs of thyroid disease. I have never learned of that many signs, but there are many.

One of the most common signs is retraction of the upper eyelids.

This is more prominent when there is proptosis (forward bulging of the eyes) that spreads the eyelids. Lid retraction may be either unilateral or bilateral. Clinical eye lid retraction is the elevation of the upper eyelid to the point that white sclera can be seen between the eyelid and the upper edge of the cornea or iris.

Movement of the upper eyelid and the eyeball may be abnormal.

On upward gaze, the eyelid may retract, but the eye will not look up. Sometimes both go up. As gaze is lowered, the eyelid may fall in a jerky, stepwise manner, rather than the usual smooth movement. Sometimes when going from up gaze to down gaze, the eyelids lag behind, exposing the upper sclera. When going from straight ahead to up gaze, the eyelid my overshoot and then drop back. The blinking rate in usually increased and proptosis of the eye may make it difficult for the eyelid to cover the front of the eyes producing the feeling of dryness and scratchy sensation.

The forward bulging of the eyes in thyroid eye disease, called exophthalmos, can involve one or both eyes. It is caused by infiltration of the extra ocular muscles by glycosaminoglycans. The affinity of the glycosaminoglycans for water causes the muscles to swell, placing pressure on the eyeball and pushing it forward.

Stretch of the optic nerve and pressure on it from the swollen muscle may cause loss of vision and glaucoma. It is important for the patient to have frequent visual field examinations during the active part of this disease to look for optic nerve damage. The optic nerve may swell and bulge as it enters the eye, because of pressure on it behind the eyeball.

The swelling of the extraocular muscles may cause limitation of up, down, right, or left gaze in one or both eyes. This may result in double vision in one or more directions of gaze including straight ahead. Muscle involvement is highly variable from only one isolated muscle to all six muscles in each eye.

When the proptosis of the eyes is great and the eyelids cannot close over the cornea, the surface of the cornea may break down and/or become infected. There is a loss of tear production and lack of blinking to spread the tears. The eye surface becomes dry and painful.

> We had a patient in Boston who had severe thyroid exophthalmos and developed a bacterial infection of one cornea and a fungal infection of the other cornea. He had scarring of both corneas to the point of legal blindness, but, because of his severe proptosis, his eyelids could not protect a corneal transplant, so it was not done.

The seven classes of eye symptoms of thyroid disease (0-6) are remembered by the acronym NO SPECS. "N" (0) is for no signs or symptoms, "O" (1) is for only eyelid signs, "S" (2) is for soft tissue involvement, i.e. swelling, "P" (3) is for proptosis greater that 22 mm, forward from the lateral orbital rim, measured by the exophthalmometer, "E" (4) is for extraocular muscle involvement, "C" (5) is for corneal involvement, and "S" (6) is for sight loss due to optic nerve involvement.

Exophthalmos is the term reserved for proptosis in thyroid disease. Thyroid disease is the most common cause of unilateral and bilateral proptosis, or exophthalmos. A tumor behind the eye is the next most common cause of unilateral proptosis.

The treatment of thyroid eye disease varies with the symptoms and severity of the problem. People with hyperthyroid disease may be treated with radioactive iodine. This iodine is concentrated in the thyroid gland where the radioactivity becomes strong enough to destroy the thyroid tissue and bring the thyroid hormones into a normal or subnormal range. After radioactive thyroid treatment, patients may have to take thyroid tablets for the rest of their lives to have normal levels of thyroid hormones to sustain life. The dosage must be carefully regulated to prevent hyper or hypothyroid symptoms.

Treatment of the hyperthyroid disease may not decrease the exophthalmos so it may need to be treated symptomatically.

Artificial tears may be sufficient to control the discomfort from decreased tears and inadequate blinking. Sewing the eyelids together at the inner and outer margins to help close the retracted eyelids, a partial tarsorrhaphy, may help, but must not be done if it will increase pressure on the eyeball to cause glaucoma.

Guanethidine eye drops can block the overactive sympathetic enervation of the upper eyelid to treat lid retractions even when there is no exophthalmos. This is usually a short term remedy

The minor elevator muscle of the upper eyelid is controlled by the sympathetic nervous system which is stimulated by hyperthy roidism, causing lid retraction. An operation to release this muscle, called the Henderson procedure, may decrease or eliminate lid retraction. (Dr. Henderson quizzed me about this procedure when I took my oral board examination. I knew about the procedure, but did not know it was named for him. I passed.)

Strabismus surgery is usually not indicated during the acute stages of the disease when there is muscle involvement, because of the transient nature of the muscle involvement. If the involvement becomes chronic, muscle surgery may help reduce a double vision problem. The swollen muscles make it difficult to judge the amount of recession needed to straighten the eyes, so finding an ophthalmologist with experience with thyroid disease is important.

When exophthalmos is severe, or there is evidence of optic nerve damage, an orbital decompression may be indicated. In this procedure, one of the walls of the orbit (eye socket) is removed to give the muscles more room to expand and thereby relieve pressure on the optic nerve.

Neurosurgeons may remove the roof of the orbit, leaving no bone between the membranes that cover the brain (meninges) and the contents of the eye socket. This allows the orbital contents to expand to relieve the pressure. The normal pulsation of the brain can be transmitted from the brain to the orbit making the eye pulsate in and out.

Removal of the floor of the orbit allows the orbital fat and inferior muscles to drop into the maxillary sinus to relieve the pressure. If he eye sinks in the socket, it may be difficult for the brain to align that eye with the other to avoid double vision.

Some surgeons prefer to remove the lateral wall of the orbit behind the temporalis muscle. The bone here is very thin so this does not add much room to the orbit. It changes the outer wall from bone to muscle which has more give and allows the muscles to expand. The same is true with removal of the nasal wall of the orbit. These orbital decompressions are often vision saving procedures.

Hypothyroid disease does not have significant eye signs other than myxedema. Myxedema includes firm edema of the skin, dry skin, hair loss, sub normal body temperature, and muscle weakness. Rarely a patient may have optic neuritis that may lead to blindness.

AIDS, ACQUIRED IMMUNODEFICIENCY SYNDROME

Acquired immunodeficiency syndrome (AIDS) is a disease caused by the HIV or human immunodeficiency virus. It is a retro virus that attacks specific white blood cells, T type lymphocytes or T-cells. These T-cells, also called CD-4 cells, are the main immune defense against infections and cancer.

People can be infected with the HIV virus without having the full-blown AIDS disease in a condition known as ARCS for Aids Related Complex Syndrome. AIDS is an advanced state of HIV infection that has advanced to the point where the patient has opportunistic infections and/or cancers. It is technically defined as when the CD-4 count is below 200 cells per micro liter.

The HIV virus affects the eyes both directly and by allowing opportunistic infections and cancers. HIV directly causes a microvascular disease that affects the retina. It can cause hemorrhages, areas of vascular nonperfusion, infarcts of the nerve fiber layer that are called cotton wool spots, vascular aneurysms, and telangiectasia (spider webs) of vessels. All of these occur in the retina. The vascular nonperfusion may cause neovascularization of the retina because of VEGF (see Age Related Macular Degeneration chapter). These changes may occur in HIV infected persons, ARCS, who do not yet have AIDS.

Cotton wool spots are one of the earliest and most common signs of HIV infection, but are not specific for HIV. They also occur in diabetes and high blood pressure. Hemorrhages can occur in different layers of the retina so they may appear round with fuzzy edges when they are deep in the retina, or flame shaped when they are in the nerve fiber layer on the surface of the retina.

Large vessels may be affected by the virus causing central retinal artery or vein occlusions that cause immediate and significant vision loss.

HIV virus can cause problems with the optic nerve. The nerve may appear swollen and pale. There may be visual loss from optic atrophy or anterior ischemic optic atrophy from vascular disease of the optic nerve. Swelling of the optic nerve head in AIDS patients may be caused by increased intracranial pressure from non Hodgkin's lymphoma, toxoplasma encephalitis, and cryptococcal meningitis that are all opportunistic infections, or cancers, in AIDS patients.

Most of the visual loss from AIDS is from opportunistic infections. These affect the eyelids, conjunctiva, cornea, retina and choroid, including the iris and ciliary body. Many of these diseases may attack immune competent patients but they are more common and progress more rapidly in AIDS patients. They may be multifocal, slow to respond to therapy, and spread to unusual tissues in the presence of the HIV virus.

Both Herpes Zoster and Herpes Simplex may be more severe in AIDS patients. Zoster, manifesting as shingles, is more likely to infect the cornea and may recur much more frequently. When shingles occurs in patients under forty-five, it is usually associated with HIV or AIDS. Herpes simplex of the skin, mucous membranes, and cornea is common in AIDS. Recurrence is more common and the duration is usually prolonged for each episode.

Because of the possibility of spreading to the brain, both herpes viruses are treated aggressively with intravenous, topical, and intraocular drugs. A slow release pellet of gancyclovir may be implanted within the eye to treat herpes infections. Recovering patients are usually advised to take oral antivirals daily to avoid recurrence. This prophylaxis is about 50% effective in preventing recurrence.

AIDS patients are very susceptible to infections with fungal organisms after minor trauma to the ocular surface. The most common organisms are from the Candida species. They are treated with antifungals, but are slower to respond when HIV is present.

Intraocular infections cause uveitis. Common causes are histoplasmosis, coccidiomycosis, toxoplasmosis, syphilis, and tuberculosis.

These organisms can infect the iris, ciliary body and the choroid. The most common symptom is photophobia, or eye pain in bright lights. These infections are treated systemically for the specific organism along with cycloplegia (paralysis of the intraocular muscles) for comfort, and steroids to combat inflammation.

Because of the sexual transmission of AIDS, it is often accompanied by syphilis, gonorrhea, and cytomegalovirus. The latter is very uncommon in immune competent people, but is a very common ocular infection in AIDS patients. Syphilis is a much more aggressive disease and requires much higher doses of medication for treatment in the presence of AIDS. Without AIDS the dose of penicillin is 2 million units, given once. In an AIDS patient, the recommended dosage of penicillin G is 12 – 24 Million units per day, repeated for a minimum of 10 days if there is ocular involvement or neuro-syphilis is suspected.

Immunocompromised patients are very susceptible to CMV (Cytomegalovirus) retinitis. It is the most common retinal infection in HIV positive patients; up to 40% of HIV positive patients will get CMV retinitis. If it is found in only one eye, it is very important to treat that eye immediately to prevent occurrence in the second eye. CMV is in the herpes family and responds to gancyclovir or foscarnet. Gancyclovir is often administered as a sustained release pellet that is inserted into the eye. CMV retinitis does not attack the healthy eye in a non compromised patient. It will attack the retina in a fetus if the mother is infected with CMV.

All of these diseases are much easier to control if they are caught early. Once large parts of the retina have been destroyed, the vision will not return. Many AIDS patients go blind before they succumb to the disease. Therefore, it is important for HIV positive patients to have frequent eye examinations by someone who is competent with the indirect ophthalmoscope. The indirect ophthalmoscope is the one that the doctor wears on his head.

There is a very bright light and a hand held, high plus lens that is held near the eye to condense the light and form a three dimensional virtual image. This instrument allows the ophthalmologist to see the entire retina and vitreous body.

Another common problem in AIDS patients is the occurrence of a particular tumor, Kaposi Sarcoma. Herpes virus has been shown to cause Kaposi Sarcoma which is extremely rare in immune competent patients but often associated with AIDS.

This is a highly vascular tumor that presents on the eyelid, and on the sclera of the eye. It forms clusters of purple-red nodules.

It can also be found in the orbit. Treatment is by local excision to keep it from becoming large enough to interfere with vision or eyelid function. Kaposi Sarcoma can occur throughout the body.

If the tumor presents a problem, it can be treated by freezing, radiation, chemotherapy or surgical excision.

Part III

EYE PROBLEMS OF CHILDREN

EMBRYOLOGY AND CONGENITAL EYE PROBLEMS

The eye is not fully developed at the time of birth. The retina does not reach a normal anatomical configuration until the child is about one-year-old. The macula and fovea are the last parts of the eye to reach their final form. Therefore, a child is not capable of sharp vision until after one year of age.

Connections with the brain, through the optic nerve, the optic tracts and the optic radiations continue to form until about the age of seven or eight years. If the eye is incapable of providing good optic nerve signals to the brain, these connections do not continue to represent the retina on the visual cortex and the representation may deteriorate.

Anything that affects the ability of the eye to see am image and transmit that image to the brain may lead to permanently poor vision, if it is not remedied before the child is seven years old. The usual causes of this poor vision are poor focus from high myopia, ptosis or drooping of the eyelid, strabismus or crossed eyes, cataract, and corneal scarring. This decrease in vision is called amblyopia but it is often referred to as a "lazy eye." This lack of equal representation of both eyes in the brain may also interfere with the coordination of the eyes to work together to produce depth perception.

Children are often born with eye problems or they may develop them during childhood. It is important to detect these problems early so that they can be corrected in time for development of normal vision and eye movements and to facilitate depth perception. Studies have shown that the appreciation of shapes and movement are learned through experience seeing vertical, horizontal, and diagonal lines and objects moving across the visual area. Blocking of vision by a cataract, corneal scar, or drooping eyelid, prevents the retina from producing these patterns and the brain's experience and future recognition of shapes and motion.

The delayed development of the macula and central vision makes it hard for the brain to align both eyes to make them "straight," but most babies manage to accomplish single vision and recognition of their mother.

An infant may appear to have crossed eyes, (turned in toward each other) or wall eyes (turned outward away from each other).

As the central vision develops, the brain learns to align the eyes so that they both look at the same thing and the child is able to fixate upon an object and follow it as it moves.

Some babies are born without the ability to align the eyes and some develop this problem from age one to five years. Others have an inborn tendency to allow an eye to drift. With time, they learn to ignore the second image from that eye, so there is no stimulus to realign the eyes. This deviation may become manifest after an illness or during stress, especially a viral disease that may have an associated encephalitis, like measles. Many infants have difficulty aligning the eye when they are very tired.

The face of the fetus is developed from several masses of embryonic tissue that migrate to fuse together. The early embryo has three layers of tissue which differentiate into the organs and tissues of the body. In general, the outside layer, the ectoderm, is the neural and skin precursor; the middle layer, the mesoderm, forms bone, muscle, vessels, and cartilage; and the inner layer the endoderm, goes on to form the gastrointestinal tract and internal organs.

During early development, several ridges form on the sides of the embryo called branchial clefts. These parts of the embryo migrate forward to the midline and fuse to form the face, including the tissues around the eyes. The mesoderm in these ridges will form structures including bones, muscles, cartilage, and the sclera and choroid of the eyeball. The ectoderm layer of the embryo forms the eyelid skin, corneal epithelium, conjunctiva, and the lens of the eye. A cyst buds from the ectoderm to form the cells of the future lens. This cyst then migrates into the optic cup that has formed from the neural ectoderm. The cyst is trapped within the optic cup as it forms the eyeball. The retina and optic nerve are formed from a stalk that grows from each side of the developing brain. The ends of the stalks form cups which become the retinas.

Nerves grow from the retina and pass along the stalk to connect with nerves at the base of the brain. These nerves radiate into the cortex of the brain, at the back of the brain, to an area called the visual cortex. These nerves contact multiple neurons in the brain to create recognizable patterns of vision. All of this differentiation and consolidation to form specific body parts is controlled by complex biochemical and genetic signals. Errors in these signals may cause improper development and errors in structures. Some of these errors may show up as defects in the eye and eyelids. Considering the complexity, there are relatively few errors in development.

> A little blond girl, about two years old, was brought to the clinic in Richmond. She was very pretty, but had unusual facial appearance. She had a very tiny nose with no nasal ridge between her eyes. She had narrow slits for the openings of her eyes because of telecanthus (the nasal corners of the eyelids are too far apart), blepharophimosis

(the width of the eyelid openings is short) and ptosis (the eye lid droops). All of these deformities together were classed as a mid-facial syndrome. She would require several plastic surgery procedures when she had grown enough to make the procedures successful.

LACRIMAL (TEARING) PROBLEMS IN CHILDREN

During development of the face, the glands that make tears and saliva are differentiated from embryonic tissue. There is a large lacrimal gland that is situated in the upper, outer quadrant of each eye socket. It develops ducts that go through the upper cul-de-sac of the conjunctiva to discharge tears on the surface of the eye under the upper eyelid. Several similar glands are clustered around the jaw and discharge saliva into the mouth through ducts from each gland. The mesoderm differentiates into hundreds of small lacrimal glands that are spread throughout the conjunctiva. These secrete tears directly onto the conjunctival surface.

The tear drainage starts when the eyelids blink to spread the tears and move them toward the nasal end of the eyelid fissure.

Two small tubes (canaliculi) begin at the edge of the upper and lower eyelids respectively near the nasal ends of the eyelids. These tubes run nasally through the eyelids and come together to form a common tube, just nasal to the point where the upper and lower eyelids fuse. This common tube dilates to form a sac or reservoir (the lacrimal sac) for the tears. From this sac, the tears drain down a tube (the nasolacrimal duct,) into the nose below the inferior turbinate ridge on the lateral wall of the nasal passage.

The canaliculi, the lacrimal sac and the nasolacrimal duct all form from an epithelial cord that is generated within the face.

This cord opens to form a tube, shortly before birth.

Absence of the lacrimal glands is very rare. Small lacrimal glands may occur, usually combined with other deformities of the ocular region, especially the eye lids and conjunctiva.

The most common tearing problem in children is in the lacrimal drainage system. The epithelial cord that runs from the eye lids to the nose should open to form a tube several weeks before birth. The opening starts at both ends and proceeds toward the middle to complete the tube. Sometimes they do not meet completely, so a thin membrane persists between the two parts of the tube, forming a lacrimal duct obstruction. This will often open spontaneously by six months after birth, if left alone. In the mean time, the blockage causes tears to collect in the eye and bacteria may grow in the lacrimal sac because it does not drain. The sac will overflow the infection into the eye as mucoid pus. Mothers notice the "goopy eye" and worry about it.

It is not good to put a child under anesthesia during the first few weeks of life, if it can be avoided. Since the tube will usually open spontaneously, without intervention, the initial treatment is usually antibiotic ointment to control the spread of the infection.

Mucous and tears will pool and cause the eye to look messy. If this spontaneously clears, the tube has opened and drainage is established. No further intervention is needed.

If the eye is still messy at the age of six months, some doctors will wrap the child in a papoose and probe the tube in the office. Other doctors prefer to have better control of the child with general anesthesia. A tiny blunt, wire probe is passed down the canaliculi, into the sac and then down the nasolacrimal duct into the nose. The doctor often feels a pop when the membrane across the tube is broken. The probe should be visualized within the nose, behind the inferior turbinate, by the surgeon, to prove that the duct is open all the way through.

If a long segment of the cord is not canalized, the probe will not pass. The child will have to wait until they are seven years old, or older, to have a surgical procedure to connect the lacrimal sac to the nose by removing some of the bony wall of the nasal cavity and stitching an opening in the lacrimal sac to the lining of the nose to create a permanent hole into the nose through which the tears can flow. This procedure is called a dacryocystorhinostomy.

Another technique is to create a hole from the corner of the conjunctiva near the nose directly into the nasal passage. To keep it open, it is necessary to place a tube stent, usually made of glass or plastic, into the hole. Some people have difficulty keeping the stent in the hole and may sneeze it across the room by accident.

There are several syndromes in which children do not make sufficient tears. They are variations of skin diseases involving anhidrosis (decreased perspiration) and decreased tearing. Some children, especially from Jewish families, may develop a familial dysautonomia which manifests as profound sweating, dry eyes, blotchy skin, hyper excitability, hypertension and general disruption of the autonomic nervous system and loss of muscle tone.

This is called Riley-Day syndrome.

OTHER CONGENITAL EYE DEFECTS

Congenital eye defects can be caused by genetic predisposition or by the influence of diseases of the mother on embryonic development. Examples of genetic problems include ptosis (drooping eyelid), aniridia (rudimentary or absent iris), abnormal eye movements, and glaucoma (high pressure in the eye). Toxoplasma infection of the mother during pregnancy may cause infection in the retina and choroid in the eye of the fetus, leaving a large central scar in the retina and poor vision in that eye. Since it is a systemic infection of the fetus, it often involves both eyes and the brain.

Rubella (three day measles) infection in the mother, during the first trimester of pregnancy, may cause many problems of development of the eye including cataract (cloudy lens), retinal damage (salt and pepper retinopathy), and microphthalmus (small eye).

Evidence of infection from various viral diseases during the first trimester of pregnancy is the observation that a zone, several layers of lens fibers in thickness, like the layers of an onion, will be cloudy or opaque in the crystalline lens, while the remainder of the lens, inside and outside of this zone, is clear. This is called a zonular cataract. This zone corresponds to the level of new lens cell development at the time of the disease. New lens fibers are laid down on the outside of the developing embryonic lens and spread toward the anterior and posterior poles of the lens, between the outside of the existing lens layers and the capsule of the lens.

The face is formed, *in utero*, from the embryonic fetal gill pouches (also called branchial buds) Failure of the embryonic branchial buds to fuse to form the eyelids may leave a gap in the eyelid called a coloboma. These may occur in one or both eyes and may be in either the upper or lower eyelid. If these are large, they must be surgically closed to protect the underlying eyeball from drying and infection. They may be associated with other malformations of the face and eyeball such as low set ears or defects in the ear cartilage.

Many children are born with a tight band of tissue in the nasal corner of the eye called the epicanthus This gives the eye an oriental appearance. Fortunately, this fold usually retracts with development of the nose bridge giving the eye a normal occidental appearance. Surgery is not indicated in most cases.

Another rare deformity is a short eyelid opening. The eyelids appear to be fused from both ends, because they did not separate properly. This shortens the opening and narrows the distance between the upper and lower eyelids. This is called blepharophimosis.

Another congenital anomaly is called telecanthus.

The nasal ends of the eyelid opening (the palpebral fissure) are anatomically normal, but they are displaced away from the nose, making the eyes appear further apart and crossed. This may be associated with other congenital anomalies of the face like abnormally shaped ears, cleft lip, and cleft palate.

Children are occasionally born with droopy eyelids or ptosis.

This may occur in one or both eyes and may be minimal, or so pronounced that the child can hardly open the eye. The eyelid usually droops about two millimeters if there is damage to the sympathetic nervous supply to the eyelid. This can occur after injury to the neck during delivery. If the levator muscle, or the levator part of the oculomotor nerve, (cranial nerve III), does not develop correctly or is damaged, the eyelid usually droops more than two millimeters. The child may lean their head backward so they are looking down to be able to peer out from under the eye lid, because they are unable lift the eyelid. When a child is born with ptosis, the horizontal fold in the upper eyelid does not develop, so the eyelid is smooth from lashes to brow. If the eyelid drops so that it usually covers the pupil, in one or both eyes, early surgery is indicated to avoid amblyopia or lazy eye.

If the pupil is blocked by the drooping eyelid, ptosis, normal vision will not develop in that eye. Representation of that eye within the brain does not develop or may decrease after the pupil becomes blocked. If the levator muscle (the muscle which opens the eye) is paralyzed, the eyelid must be suspended from the eyebrow to clear the pupil for vision. Some surgeons use a permanent suture material to lift the eyelid toward the eye brow. Others use a strip of fascia lata, a tough tissue from the leg, to suspend the eyelid from the brow. Using the child's own fascia lata will avoid any rejection of foreign tissue or substances.

If the levator muscle has partial function, a surgical procedure, called a levator resection, is done to expose the levator muscle to shorten it and reattach the muscle to the cartilage in the upper eyelid, the tarsal plate, to lift the eyelid normally. When the ptosis is only one or two millimeters, a procedure, called the Fasanella procedure, can be done from the back of the eyelid to shorten the attachment of the levator muscle to the tarsal plate.

I have seen several newborn babies who were born with a large red "birth mark" on their upper or lower eyelid. This is a capillary hemangioma that can be very small or it can involve both upper and lower eyelids and part of the face. This hemangioma tends to grow and become larger until the child is about two years old, after which it begins to shrink. It often goes away completely by the time he child is old enough to go to school.

If the tumor is small, it usually causes no visual problem, although it is often a problem for the parents, who must constantly explain it to people. If the capillary hemangioma grows large enough to pull the eyelid down, covering the pupil, amblyopia, or lazy eye, can develop. The child will require intensive treatment by the parents at a later date, to treat the lazy eye, and it could lead to permanent visual loss if it is not treated. Freezing the hemangioma with a cryoprobe usually makes it go away, leaving very little, or no, scar. Large hemangiomas may require several freezing procedures, done under anesthesia.

Children may develop a bump, or mass, beneath the skin around the eye in the areas where the embryonic buds fuse during facial formation. These bumps are usually dermoid or teratoma tumors which are clumps of embryonic tissue that were trapped in the fusion lines. This trapped tissue may differentiate into many types of tissue like skin, hair, thyroid, nerve, brain, bone, tooth, and cartilage. This tissue grows as the child grows and may become apparent at different ages depending of the size of the original trapped tissue, the type of tissue it develops into, and the ability of the surrounding tissue to accommodate it without distortion. These tumors may be mistaken for a sebaceous cyst, leading the doctor to drain them. A teratoma will continue to grow after drainage so they must be excised completely to avoid recurrence.

> When I was a resident, an eighteen-year-old man came to the clinic complaining that he had a knot under the skin of his upper eyelid near the nasal end of the lid. It had been drained twice since he was twelve years old by other doctors, but it kept coming back. I consulted one of the attending surgeons who told me that it was in a prime location for a dermoid cyst. We could feel the mass in the upper nasal part of his eye socket. It felt solid and was firmly attached to the bone of the eye socket but not to the rigid part of the eyelid. We could not feel deep enough in the socket to find the back end of the mass. The attending surgeon warned me that it could extend back in to the socket behind the eye so we should schedule the

case as an orbital exploration in case we had to dissect back in to the socket.

In the operating room, we made an incision along the rim of the socket, from the nasal end of his eyebrow to the ligament holding the nasal end of the eyelids to the nasal bone. Through this incision, we incised around the lump in the skin. We dissected around the mass and followed in back into the socket. It was attached to the nasal wall of the socket at the point where two bones met and were fused together. This confirmed the origin of the cyst as a fusion line between two buds. We dissected the cyst from the bone and freed it from surrounding tissue. When it was excised, it measured about one centimeter in diameter and two and one half centimeters long. We cut it open before sending it to pathology and found that it was full of hair. The pathologist told us that it contained skin, hair, thyroid, and cartilage.

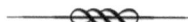

The other extreme of this occurred in a newborn black girl who was sent to the Medical College of Virginia clinic immediately after birth because one eye was bulging out so much that the eyelids would not close. My wife was the admitting intern on the pediatric ward. She called me immediately at the eye clinic to ask me to come to the ward to see this child.

The child was normal except for her face. There was a bulge in the lower eyelid on the right side that made the skin appear blue. It was pushing the eyeball up and toward the nose so much that the eyelids were separated about three millimeters when the other eye was closed.

The next day I presented her case at Grand Rounds so that all of the faculty surgeons were able to see her.

We reviewed the different types of tumors of the orbit in newborn children. Some were benign and others were malignant, such as Rhabdomyosaroma, a cancer that is rapidly fatal if it is not removed. The decision was made at the conference that we should make an incision over the tumor and remove part of it as a biopsy. If it was benign, we would remove the tumor. If it was malignant, we would remove everything from the eye socket to try to save the child's life.

Dr. Geereats, the senior full time faculty member, assisted me with the biopsy. Because of the risk involved in putting a newborn child to sleep, we had to wait for the child to be one week old before the anesthesia department would allow her to be put under anesthesia. We made an incision in the skin of the eyelid over the tumor. As soon as the skin was opened, we were looking at the tumor. It was blue-black and firm to touch. Dr. Geereats told me to cut a wedge of tissue from the tumor to send to pathology so they could tell us what kind of tissue made up the tumor.

As soon as I cut into the tissue, clear fluid gushed from the mass and it partially collapsed. We collected some of the fluid and sent it to the laboratory for analysis, because we were suspicious that it might be cerebral spinal fluid.

We left the cyst open to drain into the surrounding tissue to relieve pressure on the eyeball and decrease distortion of the face. We closed the skin and sent her back to the nursery to await the results of the biopsy and fluid analysis.

The fluid had protein, glucose and a few white blood cells, so it was consistent with cerebral spinal fluid. The biopsy contained nerves, tissue consistent with meninges (the membrane that surrounds the brain) and a tissue which looked like cerebral choroid (the tissue that makes cerebral spinal fluid in the brain). This opened the possibility that there was a hole in the cranial bone that separates the brain from the eye socket and that the meninges and part of the brain had herniated into the eye socket.

We consulted the radiologists to see if they could find the defect in the skull. This was difficult because the bones of the skull are not calcified at this age, so the bones do not show up very well on x-ray. They suggested an air pneumo-encephalogram. This test requires the injection of sterile air through the base of the skull into the meningeal sac that surrounds the brain. The air outlines the brain and meninges and will pass through a hole between the cranium and the eye socket, if it exists. They could put the baby in various positions so that the air would rise to the top and outline various parts of the brain and surrounding tissues.

They told us that they turned her every which way, but could not get the air to go into the eye socket. They could not even demonstrate a dimple where such a tract could connect to the eye socket. They were sure that there was no connection between the brain and the eye socket.

The case was presented at grand rounds again the following week for advice about what to do next. The decision was made to remove the tumor to get a definitive diagnosis. Dr. Guerry, the department chairman, was the only ophthalmologist in Richmond with much experience in orbital exploration, so he assisted me on my first orbital exploration. Because of the proposed length of the surgical procedure, we had to wait until she was three weeks old before anesthesia would put her to sleep this time.

We opened the orbit (eye socket) from the temporal side and exposed the tumor. It was below, behind, and lateral to the eyeball with the lateral rectus muscle stretched around it. We freed the tumor from the surrounding tissue very easily and found that it was attached to the bone of the eye socket. We cut the tumor from the bone and removed it. Dr. Guerry told me that it was probably not malignant because it was easy to separate from the surround tissues. He put the tumor on the mayo stand tray and cut it open. It contained clear fluid and hair and some very firm tissue which was probably non-calcified bone.

These were confirmed by the pathologist. They also found choroid tissue which was probably the source of the fluid that we released when we took the biopsy. These confirmed that it was a congenital orbital teratoma

She was in the hospital for ten days after the surgery because of a wound infection. My wife treated the infection with Gentamycin, which was so new, having been just released by the FDA, that they had to measure out each dose into a vial and add sterile water to give it to her intravenously.

When I saw her in the clinic six weeks later, her eye appeared normal, although it was turned toward her nose.

We knew that the lateral rectus muscle had been severely stretched and might not be working well enough to pull her eye straight, but that it would probably shrink with time and might become functional. If not, it could be shortened when she was older, depending on her vision.

Unfortunately, she disappeared from the clinic and was not seen again before the end of my residency. I hope that they eventually came back for continued treatment so she could see with that eye.

A review of the literature showed that this was the first reported case where a large teratoma of the eye socket, that was present at birth, was removed without also removing the eyeball. Because we had left the eyeball and the optic nerve, there is a chance that she could develop normal vision in that eye. The fear of a rhabdomyosarcoma had caused other surgeons to remove everything in the socket and then discovering that the tumor was benign. By using a biopsy to rule out a rhabdomyosarcoma, we were able to remove only the tumor and leave the eyeball, optic nerve and muscles to preserve vision.

There is another tumor called a dermoid that occurs on the surface of the eyeball. It appears as a round orange-brown, elevated mass that straddles the limbus, the transition zone between the sclera and the cornea. These can usually be shaved off when the child is old enough to be a good anesthesia risk. The area beneath the corneal portion of the dermoid does not become clear cornea, but usually remains white like the sclera. These tumors are benign so they are often left until the child wants to have it removed.

The size of the cornea at birth is usually about 10 mm in diameter. If it is less than 10 mm, the problem is called a micro cornea. This is usually accompanied by microphthalmus, meaning the whole eye is small. Microphthalmus is associated with cataract, aniridia (diminished or absent iris), glaucoma, and coloboma (congenital absence of normal eye tissue).

If the cornea is larger than 12 mm in diameter at birth, it is called megalocornea. This may be a genetic disorder or it may be secondary to congenital glaucoma. In glaucoma, the high pressure in the eye causes the infant eye to stretch, enlarging the cornea and tearing the corneal lining composed of Descemet's membrane, and the attached endothelium. Tears in this barrier layer allow the cornea to swell, become cloudy, and form a scar.

Congenital glaucoma requires immediate intervention to lower the intraocular pressure to preserve vision and prevent pain.

A child with congenital glaucoma will often exhibit aversion to light by turning the head away from light or burying their face in the pillow. Some babies with congenital glaucoma become fretful when they are in bright light, closing their eyes to avoid the light. This behavior should prompt having the child seen by an ophthalmologist.

Hazy cornea can also be caused by trauma to the cornea during birth, especially following a forceps delivery. There may be streaks on the cornea corresponding to the tears in Descemet's membrane and endothelium, caused by the forceps crushing the eye. Properly applied forceps should not press on the eye, but the obstetrician cannot see where he is placing the forceps and has to go by feel. The landmarks of the baby's skull can be confusing at that point in delivery. This infant will also show avoidance of light, like in glaucoma, because of the corneal edema. More information can be found in the chapter on glaucoma.

A child may be born with a defect in the iris which distorts the pupil. If a notch in the pupil is down and toward the nose it is probably caused by poor closure of the optic cup during the development of the eyeball. This defect in closure, called a coloboma, may also manifest as a gap in the iris, lens, retina, choroid, and/or optic nerve, inside the eye.

The iris may have more than one hole. This is known as polycoria, or multiple pupils. It is often associated with congenital glaucoma, micro cornea, and other congenital deformities. Only one of these holes is surrounded by muscles as a true pupil allowing it to dilate and constrict with changes in light or with medications.

The other holes are just defects in the iris tissue. These secondary pupils will passively change shape when the true pupil is dilated, usually contracting when the true pupil dilates and enlarging when the true pupil constricts.

A child with a white or hazy pupil probably has a cataract.

The most common cause in the past years was maternal Rubella (three day measles). Cataract from Rubella may be small and off center allowing relatively normal vision or a may be dense white blocking all useful vision. Usually this condition involves both eyes, leaving the child blind until the cataracts are removed.

Often the vision is normal after the removal of the cataract and optical correction with glasses or contact lenses, but rubella may also affect the retina, severely compromising vision, after the cataract is removed. Rubella cataracts are less common since the vaccines have been developed for Rubella.

Other viral diseases may cause cataract. These tend to be zonular in nature and may be fairly transparent. I have seen several patients with zonular cataracts, which involve only a few layers of the lens. They did well in school and passed school vision exams until the age of puberty. During the teen years, the lenses rapidly became opaque with significant visual loss. These patients usually do well after cataract surgery and have not developed amblyopia.

A child with one cataract and one normal eye will develop amblyopia in the cataract eye unless the cataract is removed at an early age. Cataract surgery in children is often associated with development of glaucoma several years later.

Cataract surgery in children is different from adult cataract removal. In the infant and young person, actually up to age 35 or 40, the back of the lens (cataract) is firmly attached to the anterior surface of the vitreous so the lens cannot be removed in one piece without removing some of the vitreous. Puling on the vitreous may tear the retina or ciliary body causing bleeding and/ or retinal detachment.

To remove the lens in a young person, the lens must be entered by cutting or tearing the capsule on the front of the lens. A large, blunt needle is introduced into the center of the lens and the soft, cortical part of the lens is aspirated completely—like sucking Jell-O through a large straw. The lens capsule is left in the eye, still attached to the vitreous face and the zonular threads. The back of the capsule is attached to the vitreous and holds it back and prevents it from coming through the pupil.

Unfortunately, in children the capsule will become cloudy or white within weeks of the cataract operation, blinding the child again. When this happens, a sharp needle is introduced through the limbal area, once the child is asleep under anesthesia, and used to slice an opening in the opacified capsule. The tension from the zonules pulls the slit open to an oval shape, big enough for good vision. An older child can sit up to the YAG laser so that the laser can be used to blow a hole in the capsule, avoiding the need for anesthesia, a sharp needle and the risk of infection. Most eye surgeons now make this tear in the capsule at the end of the procedure to remove the cataract, since opacification is inevitable.

When intraocular lenses were first introduced for cataract surgery, ophthalmologists tried to replace the optical power of the removed cataractous lens by placing the new plastic intraocular lenses in the eyes of children. This was fraught with complications.

Children have much more protein in the aqueous fluid than adults. When the eye is opened, this protein rich fluid becomes a gel, sticking to everything, especially the iris and the implanted lens. This leads to glaucoma, a dislocated lens, iris distortion and other problems.

Intraocular lenses in children soon acquired a bad name and caused their use in children to be banned. However, surgeons who operated on animals, which also have a protein rich aqueous, learned that putting heparin in the aqueous humor, before the eye was opened, prevented the gel formation and greatly reduced these complications. However, the ban on lenses in children's eyes persists in most places. I implanted several lenses in children before the ban and they worked very well. Because of my experience operating on animals, in my research, I knew to use the heparin before I placed these lenses. These small children were able to pick up small balls of paper using the vision from the implant lenses. They were usually too young to test visual acuity by standard methods.

Other causes of a white pupil include intraocular tumors such as retinoblastoma, Toxocariasis (a parasite), and retrolental fibroplasia, also called retinopathy of prematurity.

Retinoblastoma is a tumor which arises from the retina and may occur in both eyes, often spreading to the brain and orbital tissue, leading to death. It may be spontaneous or hereditary.

Adults who have survived a retinoblastoma should have genetic counseling. The treatment for the tumor is usually enucleation (removal) of the eye with the tumor to avoid spread of the tumor.

If it is bilateral, radiation or chemotherapy may be used to try to preserve vision.

Retrolental fibroplasia is also called retinopathy of prematurity (ROP). Premature infants have underdeveloped lungs and require supplemental oxygen to survive. Once the hyaline membranes that line the premature lung break up, the oxygen levels of the blood increase dramatically, especially if the infant is on supplemental oxygen.

The retinal vessels are not fully formed in a premature baby and do not extend all the way to the edge of the retina. If there is an excessive level of oxygen in the blood, the retinal vessels will form a network at the leading edge of the blood vessels on the retina. After the excess oxygen has been terminated, the vascular network forms a fibrous band around the inside of the eye on the surface of the retina. This band shrinks and pulls the retina off of the normal attachments and pulls it into a ball, behind the lens, making the pupil white.

Premature infants on supplemental oxygen must be monitored closely so that the oxygen can be discontinued immediately when the oxygen in the blood increases. This prevents the formation of the vascular network and subsequent retinal detachment. Once the vascular network has formed, it is very difficult to treat ROP.

This treatment with oxygen presents a conundrum in informed consent. If the oxygen is not used, the child will often die from lack of oxygen, but will not develop ROP if they survive. If oxygen is used, the child has a better chance of living, but may go blind later. Blood oxygen sensors are used to try to detect the exact moment when oxygen levels rise to above normal levels, but may not be monitored closely enough to decrease the oxygen levels in a timely manner.

No safe level has been determined for blood oxygen level in this situation. It appears to vary with the individual. All premature babies who were treated with oxygen must be followed by an ophthalmologist for several months after the oxygen is stopped to look for signs of the vascular network or the fibrous band developing. Treatment during the early stages of ROP is sometimes successful.

The courts have ruled that a child who was blinded by ROP after oxygen treatment for prematurity may sue the doctor for using oxygen when they become of majority age. They have two years in which to sue the doctor, even though their parents gave permission to use oxygen to save their life when they were born prematurely, knowing that the infant might become blind if they survived.

There are several congenital syndromes that cause displacement of the lens, including Marfan's Syndrome and Marchesani's syndrome. Marfan's syndrome is characterized by long bones, especially fingers and toes, relaxed ligaments, deformities of the spine, and heart disease. Marchesani's syndrome children are short and have spade shaped hands and feet. They have a type of glaucoma that is very hard to control and often leads to blindness.

Children with these syndromes should be examined frequently by an ophthalmologist.

Other congenital disorders can change the shape of the lens (anterior and posterior lenticonus and Alport's syndrome). These lens problems can be treated with glasses or cataract extraction, depending of the particulars of the case. If the lens is pulled off center by the disease, the patient may use cataract glasses or contact lenses to see around the cataract. These lenses are very strong because the lens is not in the axis so that the lens power must be replaced. If the lens is displaced but not far enough to see around, the lens can be removed and the child treated with a contact lens and intermittent patching of the other eye to avoid amblyopia.

Children are sometimes born with very thin sclera, the tough, white, outer coating of the eye. The dark choroid shows through the thin sclera, giving a light blue color to the sclera. This blue color usually disappears during the first few weeks of life making the sclera very white.

If the sclera has a persistent blue color, it may be that the child has the genetic disorder called osteogenesis imperfecta, in which the child has a deficiency in forming bones. The bones are very fragile and cause the child to have repeated bone fractures and arrested development. Blue sclera can also occur in Marfan's syndrome, pseudoxanthoma elasticum, and Ehlers-Danlos syndrome (rubber man syndrome). Children with osteogenesis imperfecta may develop keratoconus, megalocornea, and cataracts.

ACQUIRED EYE PROBLEMS IN CHILDREN

The major problems that most pediatric ophthalmologists see in their offices are with children whose eyes that do not work well together. However, there are many other problems that occur mostly in children. Although some of these problems are present at birth, most of them occur during the first few years of life. Some of the problems may go undetected until the teens or later.

When a child is born with a red, swollen eye and a purulent (pus) discharge, or this discharge develops within the first two weeks of life, the infection is called neonatal ophthalmia. There are specific causes for these infections and the time of onset is often helpful in determining the applicable cause.

All babies who are born in a hospital must have a prophylactic treatment for ocular syphilis and gonorrhea within twenty-four hours of birth. The standard treatment in most hospitals in the past was eye drops of 1% silver nitrate in each eye. Silver nitrate will kill the spirochetes of syphilis and the bacteria that cause gonorrhea and most other bacteria. These infections were common before the modern treatments for these diseases were developed and women began having long term prenatal care. Silver nitrate 1% eye drops, known as Crede prophylaxis are still given in hospitals today, although many hospitals now use erythromycin ointment instead.

Ocular discharge that appears on the first or second day of life is usually a reaction to the silver nitrate or antibiotic given at birth. After that time, bacterial conjunctivitis may be caused by common bacteria in the birth canal such as staphylococcus. These bacteria may spread from parts of the baby's body that were not treated by the Crede prophylaxis. This type of infection is treated by appropriate antibiotics.

If the eyes are quiet until ten to fourteen days after birth and then become inflamed, the cause is probably Chlamydia, acquired in the birth canal. This is effectively treated with either tetracycline ointment or sulfacetamide eye drops. Tetracycline should not be given systemically to children because it damages their bones and teeth, even non erupted teeth.

Several states are now trying to legislate that every child born in a hospital must have an eye examination before they are allowed to leave the hospital. When I was an intern on obstetrics, it was our responsibility to give each baby a complete newborn physical exam, including an eye exam, within 24 hours of delivery.

That may have been the luxury of having interns and residents working in the hospital. When my father practiced general medicine and delivered babies, each new baby was a new patient for him, to look after and assume their medical care. He made sure that they had a thorough examination as soon as the mother was able to leave the delivery suite.

Strabismus

First, let me define some terms. Strabismus is a state of lack of parallelism of the visual axes of the eyes. Some people refer to this as squint. A phoria is a latent deviation of the eyes that is held in check by binocular vision. The eyes are usually straight, but deviate when the child is tired or sick. A tropia is a manifest deviation of the eyes that is not controlled by binocular vision.

The eyes are not aligned, either crossed or turned out all of the time. There are cases of intermittent tropias that go in and out of control by fusion of the images of the two eyes.

A phoria occurs when the eyes can be used simultaneously and can fuse the images from the two eyes to form one image in three dimensions (with depth perception). The brain wants to fuse the images to make one picture. When the child is tired or sick, the brain gives up trying to fuse the images and lets one eye wander.

The muscles in the eyes usually are relaxed with some muscle tone when the eyes are pointing straight ahead and looking at the same object. If they naturally want to turn in or out, they will do so when the patient is too tired or sick to fuse them by aligning the eyes, but the eyes return to straight with concentration or rest.

Tropias can be crossed, called e*S*otropia, or turned out (wall eyed), called e*X*otropia, or one eye higher that the other, called hyp*ER*tropia, and named after the higher eye, i.e. right hypertropia is the correct term when the right eye looks above the left eye.

Some people also use the term hyp*O*tropia, named after the lower eye. The standard is to use hypertropia, unless the pathology is all involving the lower eye such as with an orbital fracture entrapping the inferior rectus muscle of the involved eye, holding the eye down, producing a hypotropia of that eye. The same terminology applies for phorias: esophoria, exophoria, and hyperphoria.

There are several types of crossed eyes, or esotropia. There is congenital, or infantile esotropia which is seen within six months after the child is born. It can involve only one eye which always looks toward the nose or it can alternate with each eye deviating while the other looks at the mother or something that attracts the baby's attention.

I have had mothers tell me that they think that their child is cross eyed. They usually say that they notice it when they are nursing the baby. Many children have extra skin in the nasal end of the upper eyelid because the nose is not well developed.

When the child looks up at their mother while they are nursing, they usually look to one side, toward the mother. This movement hides one eye behind this lax upper eyelid, making the child look cross-eyed. As the child grows, the skin will be retracted by the ridge of the nose, showing more of the sclera (white of the eye) on the nasal side of the eye and the child's eyes will appear straight.

When I test the eyes of this child, I use a point source of light like a pen light. I hold the light in front of the child, about a foot away from the eyes, and try to attract the baby's attention to the light by movement or flashing. The light will be reflected as a single spot of light on the front of each eye. If both eyes are looking at the light, the spot will be near the center of the pupil, slightly nasal to the center, symmetrically in both pupils. If one eye is looking at the light and the other is not, the point of light will be near the center of the pupil of the eye that is looking at the light and not within the pupil in the other eye. How far from the center depends on how much the second eye is deviated,

If only one eye deviates all of the time, it may mean that the child cannot see well with the deviated eye and needs to have a complete eye exam to determine if that is the case and why.

Cataracts, intraocular infections, and ocular tumors are causes of this type of esotropia. When deviations occur from poor vision in one eye after the child is seven years old, the eye often turns out rather than inward.

> When I was a second year resident, I was called by a pediatric resident and asked to see a child with crossed eyes. I was on the strabismus service, so I agreed to see her right away. When she sat in my exam chair, I saw immediately that she had severely crossed eyes. I tried to measure the amount that they crossed, but found that the amount of crossing varied from measurement to measurement. When I refracted her for glasses, I found that she was about +2.00 Diopters farsighted in each eye.

That was before I put any eye drops in her eyes. After I put eye drops in her eyes to block all of her accommodation (focusing), she needed +4.00 Diopters in each eye. I made up some glasses with trial frames and the loose lens set and put them on her.

Voila! She was straight. I told her parents that we should order glasses for her to make her straight. Her mother told me that she had been seen by a "Pediatric Optometrist" who was ordering glasses for her.

I knew that optometrists in Virginia were not allowed to use medications, including eye drops, so he would not know that she needed a full +4.00 Diopters in each eye to make her straight. I decided to call him to tell him the full amount of farsightedness that I had uncovered with the drops so that the glasses would be strong enough to make her straight.

Many children develop esotropia when they are two or three years old or older. This esotropia tends be worse when the child is tired, or not feeling well. It could be described as wobbly in the amount of crossing. This type of esotropia is caused by the fact that the child is very far sighted and must focus their vision nearer, just to see at distance.

There is neurological reflex of combined movements called the synkinetic near response. When the eye focuses closer (accommodation), the eyes also turn inward to look at a near object (accommodative convergence), and the pupil becomes smaller (miosis), which increases the depth of focus. When these farsighted children focus in, their eyes turn in automatically. Usually one stays on the target and the other turns in toward the nose.

Once the eye has turned in, vision turns off in the brain so the child does not see double. This removes all stimulus for the eye to align itself with the other eye. The longer the crossing persists, the more vision tends to turn off and the harder it is for the child to align the eyes. If one eye turns off all of the time, it may become lazy.

Fortunately, this type of esotropia, the kind the little girl had, called accommodative esotropia, is easy to treat in the early stages. It requires correcting the farsightedness with glasses.

Treating the farsightedness removes the need to focus at distance so the eyes do not cross. In most children, the focusing to see at near turns the eyes in the appropriate amount so that both eyes are looking at the same place and the eyes are working together, fusing, all the time. In some children, especially after they have had accommodative esotropia for a while, they develop some esotropia that is not corrected by the glasses. This either means that the glasses are not strong enough or that they have developed a residual esotropia.

To be sure that the glasses are strong enough, the measurement of farsightedness must be done with eye drops to completely paralyze the accommodation. Most ophthalmologists will use atropine ointment, given two or three times a day for three days by the mother, before the measurement for glasses.

The nice thing about using atropine is that it lasts about three weeks. The measurement for glasses, (refraction), is done and the glasses are ordered immediately. When they are delivered within two weeks, the child still cannot focus to see without the glasses because of the residual effect of the atropine. When the glasses are placed on the child's face, they smile and want to wear the glasses, because they can see again. If they are allowed to regain their ability to accommodate (focus), they will be focusing all of the time. They will add the habitual focusing to power to the glasses and the glasses will be too strong. When they try to focus, the eyes will turn in again. Without the use of atropine, they must wear the new glasses for two to three weeks to learn not to focus. Meanwhile, the vision will be blurred and there will be a struggle for the mother to keep the glasses on the child.

Back to the little girl: Unfortunately, when I called the "pediatric optometrist" he was very condescending and told me that he knew better than any resident in training what to do for the child. He told me that he used fixation with movie cartoons to relax all accommodation and that she would never tolerate the full +4.00 Diopter correction.

Movies do not relax the habitual accommodation which is used to see at distance. A far sighted person has to focus some to see the movie on the screen. That part of focusing would not be measured.

He told me that these children are brain damaged and never become completely straight. He said that he would start the child wearing the frames without lenses to get them used to the frames. Then, after two or three weeks, he would put +0.50 lenses in the frames for three months for her to get used to a small amount of correction. Then every three months he would increase the power by 0.50 Diopters until he reached the full +2.00 in both eyes.

He knew that she would still not be straight and that she might accept some more power in the lenses later. I knew that this is because she would be under corrected for straightening the eyes and still be focusing. Once part of the farsightedness is corrected, the child would relax some of the habitual focusing and would accept more correction.

He did not say that meanwhile he has sold four pairs of lenses to the girl's parents.

I knew that she would be straight if she had a full correction. She had demonstrated that in my exam chair that day. Since he did not use eye drops, he had probably not experienced what a full correction would do. Since he never fully corrected the problem, his children were never straight, so he probably believed they were brain damaged.

I tried to argue with him, but he told me that I did not know what I was talking about, so I should send her back to him.

I explained to the parents that I would order different glasses for their child that would work better than the other "eye doctor's," but they told me that they had already paid for the glasses and spent more than they could afford for the eyeglasses from the optometrist. They had no more money to buy more glasses. I knew that I would be facing legal problems if I tried to discredit the optometrist, so I left it alone for the parents to decide. They disappeared from my office and did not return. In most states, optometrists can now use eye drops for refraction and should, by now, have learned to treat this condition correctly.

A few of the children with accommodative esotropia will be straightened with glasses at distance, but still cross when looking at something close to them. This happens when the synkinetic near response is not correct. These children will cross their eyes more than they should for the amount of accommodation (focusing) that they use. This crosses the eyes at near. This type of esotropia is called high AC/A ratio esotropia (Accommodative Convergence to Accommodation ratio). To treat this we must decrease the amount that the eyes focus for near. To decrease the amount of focusing the eyes do, we can add more plus correction for near, by using a bifocal lens in the glasses. To teach the child to use the bifocal lens, looking through the top half for distance and the bottom half for near, we line up the horizontal dividing line of the lens at the middle of the pupil.

Another type of esotropia is called alternating esotropia. The child can see with both eyes, but they use only one at a time, allowing the other to turn in toward the nose. If someone approaches from their right, the left eye has a tendency to look that way so they watch the person with their left eye. If the person walks past them, they may switch to the right eye as the person passes.

They do the reverse if something approaches from the left. They may look straight ahead with one eye and blink, changing to look at the same object with the other eye with the first eye turned inward. This is called alternate fixation. These children usually maintain good vision in both eyes and do not develop amblyopia, or lazy eye.

Children can benefit from surgery to straighten the eyes so they can easily look at the same object with both eyes simultaneously, some can learn to fuse the images in the brain to get depth perception. Many of these patients do not learn to fuse the images for depth perception but can hold their eyes straight. The brain may use large objects in the images from both eyes to align the images and therefore align the eyes. Some will drift back to esotropia or may develop exotropia instead and need further surgery to straighten the eyes again at the age when they become very image conscious, during puberty.

Some esotropia is because of one eye is very out of focus, either from nearsightedness or farsightedness. This is called refractive esotropia. The crossed eye cannot focus on an object at the same time the other eye is focused on it. Therefore that eye has blurred vision all of the time. As the dominant eye focuses at near, the other eye is out of focus. Both eyes always focus the same amount so when the dominant eye changes focus, so does the blurred eye, remaining blurred. The brain soon learns to ignore the blurred picture which is competing with the other eye for recognition by the brain. This makes the out of focus eye lazy (amblyopic).

To correct this problem, the vision in both eyes must be optimized with glasses or contact lenses. If the bad eye is very different in focus, (myopia or hyperopia) a contact lens must be used to minimize the difference in image size caused by the difference in optical powers needed to correct the two eyes. This can be a problem in children, but most pediatric ophthalmologists employ specialists to facilitate the contact lens fitting to obtain longer wearing times.

Once the lazy eye has the correct focus, the other eye must be patched to force the brain to recognize the image from the lazy eye and allow that eye to become better represented in the brain.

This may take weeks or months. The child must use the good eye part of the time so that it does not become lazy under the patch.

Intermittent patching may have to be continued until the child is seven or eight years old to avoid the recurrence of amblyopia.

Testing for ocular alignment

When a card, or occluder, is placed over one eye, the child is forced to look, or fixate, with the eye that is not covered. The other eye, the vision being blocked, may turn in or out behind the cover. This is called cover testing. It is used to text for tropias and phorias. If the deviated eye stays deviated when the cover is removed, it shows that the eye has been turned off (suppressed) and does not realize that it is deviated. This is a tropia. If the deviated eye returns to straight as soon as it is uncovered, it was not turned off or suppressed. This is a phoria.

When the occluder is moved rapidly to cover one eye and then the other eye, the previously deviated eye will now look at the fixation target while the formerly fixing eye will turn out behind the cover. This is called alternate cover testing. It will detect latent phorias.

If one eye is covered and the covered eye is allowed to turn in or out and then the cover is removed so that both eyes can look at the fixation target, the eye may stay deviated, or it may snap back so that both eyes are looking that the fixation target.

If the deviated eye snaps back, the child has exophoria. A phoria is a tendency for the eyes to deviate but not to turn off, or suppress.

When the deviating eye remains deviated after the cover is removed, it means that the eye was turned off when it deviated.

This is called exotropia. The term tropia is used when the deviated eye does turn off, or suppresses.

The eye that deviates may be partially turned off so there is no double vision to make the brain line up the deviated eye. Once the eye is deviated and turned off, it may also turn up or down depending on which rotating muscle is dominant. This condition may be intermittent or constant. The longer this problem exists, the greater the deviation may become. Phorias my become tropias.

Fortunately, in exotropia, the suppression of the brain for the deviated eye involves only half of the retina. This is the outer half of the retina from the fovea toward the temporal side of each eye. The image that the fixating eye sees straight ahead, centered in the vision, would be seen by the temporal retina in the other eye. Since the temporal retina is suppressed, the child does not see double.

If the eyes are surgically straightened to a slight over correction, the brain will see double from the overlapping of the vision in the nasal half of the eyes. The brain will try to straighten the eyes to make a single picture, or fusion. Since the eyes now want to cross from the over correction, the double vision is from the non-suppressed retina and brain. If the eyes drift at all from straight, they go into double vision which the brain corrects by realigning the eyes.

Unfortunately, the suppression in esotropia involves a round or oval area all around the fovea, so the over correction of crossed eyes does not have the same mechanism for fine tuning the position of the eyes. It is much harder to get crossed eyes permanently straight. Usually, if the eyes that had esotropia are almost straight, the brain can use fusion of the peripheral vision to align the eyes while the central vision is still suppressed. This is called battleship fusion. They may not be able to fuse small objects, but they can make one image of something as large as a battleship.

Amblyopia can occur after surgery to straighten the eyes. If one eye is not directed to the object that is being seen, even by a few degrees, and appears to be working with the other eye, it will suppress to avoid double vision. The suppression will cause a lazy eye if the regimen of patching that eye is neglected.

I was told by one patient in Richmond that someone had told them that if they got their eyes straightened, one eye would go blind. This person had alternating esotropia and was a candidate for surgery, but would have to be watched for amblyopia after surgery.

These children with esotropia rarely get stereoscopic vision or depth perception after surgery. Depth perception requires that the brain is receiving simultaneous images from both eyes. The images are slightly different because of the separation of the eyes by the nose. The brain uses the differences in the two images to construct a view that has separation of the objects by distance, or in three dimensions.

Once an eye has deviated, in or out, fusion is lost and one eye is usually suppressed. Since there is no image going to the brain from the deviated eye, the brain has no control over where it turns. It will often point upward or downward depending on the pull of the other muscles that move the eye.

There are many secondary deviations and patterns of crossed eyes that are best determined by an experienced ophthalmologist.

Pediatric ophthalmologists specialize in this type of problem.

I cannot over emphasize the importance of avoiding amblyopia or lazy eye. When an eye deviates and is suppressed, the representation of the retina of that eye in the brain becomes jeopardized.

With continued suppression, the neuronal representation in the occipital cortex of the brain, decreases for that eye and the sharpness of vision decreases. This may cause severe visual loss which increases with time. If a lazy eye persists until the child is seven or eight years old, it will become permanent, because the eye looses the ability to regain representation in the brain. Before the age of seven, the eye can force representation in the brain again, if the amblyopic eye is used and the other eye is blocked. This is done by putting an eye patch over the good eye, forcing the child to use the lazy eye. This procedure is called patching, or occlusion therapy.

If the patching is done continuously on the good eye, it can lose representation in the brain so patching must be done with care to allow the good eye to function part of the time so that it does not become lazy while the lazy eye is being treated.

Covering the good eye of a child and forcing the use of blurred vision is not something that most children will tolerate. They will usually try to remove the patch until they become accustomed to it. The first few days of patching, a parent must be present to be insistent that the patch be replaced immediately, every time it is removed. Winning this battle for the first few days is crucial if the treatment is to be successful. The child will usually accept the patch after the first few days and will not try to remove it after that.

When one eye is deviated most of the time, but not suppressed, a phoria, the child may adapt to the problem by turning their head a particular direction all of the time. This will either cause the pictures from the two eyes to come closer to alignment and allow the child to fuse the images or it will move the images farther apart so there is less optical confusion of the two images for the brain, so the brain can ignore the deviated image.

If the right eye is deviated outward, toward the right, the child will turn their head to the left. Now both eyes will look to the right and the images will be closer together. If one eye turns down, the child will tilt their head back, so both eyes will look down and possibly fuse the images from the two eyes.

When the oblique muscles are involved, the head turns become more complex like chin down (superior oblique muscle under action) and to the right (right medial rectus under action), or chin up and to the right (right inferior oblique under action).

Since the oblique muscles rotate the eye, the child may also tilt the head to the side to rotate the good eye to align with the rotated eye with the problem. If both eyes had oblique muscle problems, the turning and tilting compensations become more complex.

> Not all head turns are from strabismus. An eight-year-old, very blond boy was brought in to see me because he did not pass the school eye exam. When he sat in the exam chair, his mother told him to sit up straight, which he did.
>
> I checked his vision and he could only see about 20/80 in each eye. He told me he could make it better if he tilted his head to the left. I checked him that way and he read about 20/30.
>
> He had very light colored irises and his pupils showed a slightly pink tint to them. When I looked in his eye, the retina looked pink, rather than the usual orange. I could see some of the vessels of his choroid, showing through the retina, because he did not have any pigment behind the retina and in the choroid as he should have. I concluded that he had albinism. He had good vision for someone with albinism, because some albinos do not develop the fovea completely, leaving them with permanently decreased vision. The strange thing was that it improved when he tilted his head to the left.

I have seen several people who have high astigmatism with the axis vertical, exactly at ninety degrees. This squeezes the letters on the chart around a vertical axis, but it does not distort them very much. When the astigmatism is oblique to the vertical axis, the distortion is much worse. I checked him for astigmatism and found that he had over four Diopters (a lot) of astigmatism at 45 degrees in both eyes. Usually astigmatism is symmetrical— one eye at 45 degrees and the other at 135 degrees. Since his axes were parallel, he could tilt his head 45 degrees to make his astigmatism vertical. Once he had glasses to correct his astigmatism, he did not have to tilt his head to see 20/30.

Surgery to straighten children's eyes

Some problems with ocular alignment can be corrected with glasses or exercises, but many do not respond to these types of correction. Most eyes that are out of alignment must be straightened surgically. This is usually done by removing one or more muscles from the eyeball and moving them forward or backward to straighten the eye.

Eye muscles usually act in pairs. If the medial rectus muscle contracts, the lateral rectus muscle will relax. At the same time, the lateral rectus muscle in the other eye will contract to move both eyes in the same direction. However, if the eyes try to look at a near object, they must converge. Both eyes move toward the nose. This requires both medial rectus muscles to contract simultaneously to pull the eyes toward each other. Similar combinations exist for the oblique muscles so that the eyes can follow moving objects.

With these complex combinations of contracting and relaxing muscles, it is best to think of straightening the eyes as realigning each eye within the group of muscles that move each eye.

If the eyes are crossed, the medial rectus muscles in both eyes are removed from the sclera and reattached to the sclera a fixed distance behind the original attachments. This procedure is called a bimedial recession. This moves the pupils of the eyes away from the nose. The amount of crossing determines the distance the muscles should be recessed on the eye.

If the eyes are severely crossed, it may be necessary to also move the lateral rectus muscles forward to further rotate the eyes.

The muscles cannot actually be moved forward, so they are shortened and reattached to the same region from which they were removed. When two muscles in the same eye are moved to correct the alignment, it is called a recess and resect procedure. For extremely crossed eyes, it may be necessary to do a recess and resect procedure in both eyes.

There was a very pretty, black, high school girl in Montserrat who wanted to be a movie star. She told us that she had a lead part in the school play that was to be given in three weeks. Her eyes were crossed so much that when she looked straight ahead with one eye, the other looked at the bridge of her nose. We did a maximum recess and resect procedure in both eyes. The next day she looked perfectly straight. She was the happiest girl on Montserrat.

Six weeks later we received a letter from her saying that she had graduated from high school and planned to leave Montserrat to pursue acting school.

Strabismus Surgery Procedures

Surgery is always frightening to children so it is done under general anesthesia. Once the child is asleep, the eyelids are washed with surgical soap and the conjunctiva is rinsed with balance salt solution. An incision is made through the conjunctiva between the muscles, but near to the muscle to be operated. A muscle hook is inserted through this incision and passed underneath the muscle to be moved. The conjunctival incision is pulled over the muscle to expose the muscle where it is attached to the eyeball.

The muscle is attached to ligaments that surround it and hold it in position. These ligaments are stripped from the muscle to free it. For a recession procedure, sutures are placed in the edges of the muscle with locking stitches where it attaches to the eye.

The muscle is then cut from the eye as close to the eye as possible, without cutting the sclera, and being careful not to cut the sutures that now hold the end of the muscle. The desired amount of recession is marked on the sclera behind the original insertion with calipers. Tiny needles on the sutures in the muscles are passed through the sclera at the marked point, running just below the surface, to attach the muscle at the new, recessed, location.

This allows the eye to move away from the recessed muscle.

In the resection procedure, the sutures are placed in the edge of the muscle behind the place where it attaches to the eye. The distance behind the attachment, or insertion, of the muscle is measured carefully to give a precise amount of resection. Once the sutures are placed, a clamp is applied across the muscle just forward of the sutures to stop any bleeding in the muscle when the muscle is cut across the crush line. The stump of muscle is removed from the insertion without cutting the sclera where the muscle was attached. The muscle is then sewn to the original insertion of the muscle with the preplaced suture, thereby shortening the muscle and pulling the eye toward the resected muscle.

Similar procedures can be used to move the oblique muscles to correct over action or under action of those muscles. Some ophthalmologists treat over action of the superior oblique muscles by locating the part of the muscle tendon that goes through a ring at the upper, inner corner of the eye socket and then to the top and back of the eyeball. They bring that tendon part of the muscle forward, using a special muscle hook. They strip away the muscle sheath and cut the tendon, letting it go. This has the same effect as lengthening the muscle. This procedure is called a tendon sheath tenotomy.

> When I was in training, it was rumored that one of the eye surgeons in town had a special, three snip operation to straighten children's eyes. The procedure was so fast, that he did not use general anesthesia. The child with crossed eyes was tied to a chair and given eye drops to numb the eyes. The back of the chair was tilted back to an assistants lap while the assistant held the child's head. A speculum was placed in the eye to hold it open. Numbing eye drops were placed in the eye for anesthesia. The surgeon grasped the conjunctiva, over the muscle with forceps and made one big snip, opening the

conjunctiva. He then grabbed the fibrous tissue that was exposed, called Tenon's capsule, and made a snip through it, exposing the muscle. He then grabbed the muscle with forceps and made the third snip, cutting completely across the muscle, letting it retract.

Then he did the same procedure in the other eye. The next day the child looked much straighter than before the surgery, sometimes almost perfect.

He could get away with this imprecise surgery, because the check ligaments that were still attached to the muscle would not let it retract very much. Even if the child's eyes were still crossed, they were much straighter and the parents were usually very pleased with the result. Modern procedures are much more precise and allow a much more predictable and accurate outcome, but they take longer.

The blood supply to the front of the eye is delivered by seven arteries; these arteries come to the front of the eye through the rectus muscles. There are two arteries in each of the medial, superior and inferior rectus muscles and only one artery in the lateral rectus muscles. Removal of one muscle does not compromise the blood supply, because these arteries anastomose in a ring around the front of the eye. However, removal of two adjacent muscles may cause acute necrosis (death) of parts of the iris and ciliary body. This leads to inflammation, cataract formation, corneal edema, and atrophy of the iris and ciliary body. This complication is called anterior segment necrosis. In severe cases, this can lead to loss of the eye. Strabismus surgeons are well aware of this problem so it is a rare complication.

If the ocular alignment problem has both horizontal and vertical components, the horizontal part is treated in one eye and the vertical part is treated in the other eye so that two adjacent muscles are not removed in the same eye. If the horizontal component is too great to be corrected with one eye and requires surgery on three or four muscles, the eyes are allowed to heal and reestablish a blood supply before another procedure is done to repair the vertical problem.

Nystagmus

A few children are born with eyes that move constantly, searching randomly. Others acquire a jerking motion in their eyes by the time they are two or three years old. This motion is called nystagmus.

Adults can acquire nystagmus with neurologic disorders.

There are several kinds of nystagmus.

Nystagmus occurs normally when someone watches a train go by. The eyes follow the train briefly and they jump ahead to watch it go by again. This has one slow movement to follow the train and one fast movement to jump ahead.

People who are tired, intoxicated, or toxic on drugs will show this movement when they are asked to look far to one side and hold that position. If the examiner has the person follow a light from straight ahead to far right or left, the eyes will jerk back and forth near the periphery.

Wandering, searching nystagmus in a child, where the eyes wander back and forth, usually means that the child cannot see well. Children with opaque corneas or cataracts will usually develop nystagmus by the time they are two years old.

A child who is born with rapidly moving eyes that drift in one direction and then jerk back has congenital jerk nystagmus. This may interfere with vision and is very bothersome to the parents.

The child may develop a head turn, because there may be one direction of gaze (one position for the eyes) in which the jerking is minimal and the vision is best. This is called the null point. This point can be anywhere. It may be nearly straight ahead, or it may be far to the right or left. The ideal place for it to be is straight ahead. There is a surgical procedure wherein the muscles of both eyes are moved to rotate both eyes in the same direction, hoping to move the null point to straight ahead.

There are other rare forms of nystagmus which are best sorted out by a neuro ophthalmologist.

PINK EYE OR CONJUNCTIVITIS

One thing that will send panic through a school is an outbreak of pink eye. There are several causes for pink eyes in children. The classic cause is either Hemophilus Egyptius or pneumococcus bacteria. The conjunctiva becomes pink or red and there is a white or yellow discharge. This type of pink eye is easily spread; from eye to hand to eye, and from one person to another by contact, so schools may have to be shut down to stop an epidemic. Antibiotics are effective against bacteria.

Another common form of pink eye is caused by adenoviruses. This form is very contagious and there is no effective medication to stop the infection. It must run its course for one to two weeks and go away. During the time of infection, including the two week long asymptomatic incubation period, the disease is very contagious so infected people should not share towels, make up, or have intimate contact while the eyes are red. The disease may spread from one eye to the other causing first one eye to be red followed by the other eye becoming red two weeks later, making the disease last for four weeks. Schools may require the child to stay home until both eyes are completely white again. The eyes are infectious until all inflammation is gone. Because the eyes do not become red for about two weeks after the person is exposed, the disease is often spread widely before it is recognized.

Several years ago, there was an epidemic in Detroit. A whole assembly line was shut down because the roller towel in the restroom was jammed, so everyone wiped their hands on the same two feet of the roller towel. Most people touch their eyelids many times a day.

Other forms of conjunctivitis are caused by many other bacteria (staphylococcus, or streptococcus, Chlamydia (Trachoma) viruses (adenovirus and herpes), tick borne rickettsia (Rocky Mountain spotted fever), fungus (Candida), parasites (Trichinella), or allergies (dust or pollens).

Many childhood viral diseases such as measles, chicken pox, and mumps can cause red eyes. There may be inflammation of the cornea, causing light sensitivity which is relieved by darkening the sick room. Mumps, which usually involves the salivary glands, may cause swelling of the lacrimal (tear producing) glands in the eye socket. These glands are very similar to the salivary glands.

There are various diseases that may cause a child to be born blind, or partially sighted. If the mother has her first attack of toxoplasmosis in the third trimester of pregnancy, the organism may cross the placenta and infect the eyes and brain of her unborn child. This causes a large scar in the middle of the retina in one or both eyes, along with optic atrophy.

Toxoplasmosis is often carried by cats. There was an epidemic of Toxoplasmosis among pregnant women in Paris in the 1960's.

The epidemiologists were trying to determine whether pregnancy increased the susceptibility to the organism or the increase was because pregnant women in Paris tend to stay home with their cats. I have never learned the conclusion of this study.

Rubella (three day measles) in the first trimester of pregnancy can infect the eyes of the unborn child causing cataracts, retinopathy, and glaucoma and may lead to nystagmus later.

A two month old infant boy was brought to see me to determine whether he could see. His mother had noticed that he did not seem to look at or follow people or objects although his eyes did move together. I examined him and could not get him to look at my flashlight or follow hand puppets or flashing lights with his eyes. His retinas looked normal and there were no cataracts or corneal edema to block his vision. His pupils did constrict when a bright light was shown in to his eyes. This confirmed that the retina was working and the optic nerve and tracts were functioning as far as the base of the brain where the pupil reactions connect with the optic pathways. This did not prove that he could see.

I scheduled an electroretinogram (ERG) and visual evoked response (VER) under anesthesia for the child.

The ERG tests whether the impulse created by the rods and cones in response to light is conducted all the way to the occipital cortex which is the visual part of the brain.

The day before the ERG, the mother called me to say that she thought the child had begun to look at his hands. She said that he would throw up his right hand to the right of his face and turn to look at it. At the same time he would extend his left leg.

We started to record the electroretinogram when the child was just barely under anesthesia. The pattern of the ERG was unusual. The normal pattern is for the wiggly lines from the background noise to show a series of spikes, for the rods and cones, milliseconds after a light is flashed into the eyes. The visual evoked response shows a single spike in the occipital cortex about 540 milliseconds after the light flashes in the eye. We saw widespread spike activity before we began flashing the light. This meant that the child was having a seizure. The anesthesiologist deepened the anesthesia level and the spike activity level disappeared. Anesthesia is one way to break a seizure. We were able to record the ERG and he VER once the seizures had stopped.

The pediatric neurologist came to the operating room and examined our recordings and decided that the child had been in status epilepticus (a continuous epileptic seizure) and that the seizure condition had blocked his reaction to visual stimuli. They started the child on seizure medicine which broke the status. He began to fixate on objects and follow them with his eyes, proving that he could see them.

When the mother thought that the child was looking at his hands, he was having "Jack knife" seizures. The child throws up a hand to one side and turns their head toward it. At the same time, they extend the opposite leg. This is a distinct form of seizure.

Children are usually not aware of when they are seeing with both eyes or with only one eye. They do not complain when they lose depth perception because one eye is not seeing. This problem is usually noted by an adult, usually the mother, who notices some unusual behavior or appearance of the eyes.

When an eye drifts away from straight, it can be from weakness in aligning the eyes or from the child being unable to see with one eye, so that the brain does not have a picture from that eye to align with the image from the other eye. Any child with an eye that drifts from straight ahead should be examined by a physician to determine whether there is some reason that the child is not seeing in the deviating eye. There can be a tumor in the eye or a destructive lesion of the retina or choroid that has damaged the central vision in the eye. If the child has a cataract, it may distort the vision so that the brain cannot align the eyes.

One sign that should be investigated immediately is the appearance of a white pupil. Normally the pupil is black because there is not enough reflected light from the retina to light up the pupil. If there is a tumor or a parasitic worm in the eye, or a retinal detachment, the white surface of that object will cause the pupil to appear white. A dense cataract will also cause a white pupil. These are all serious problems which must be addressed immediately to save vision and possibly save the life of the child.

HEREDITARY DISEASES IN CHILDREN

D iseases that may become apparent during childhood that are hereditary in nature are most commonly caused by either metabolic malfunctions or connective tissue diseases.

The most common connective tissue diseases in children are Marfan's and Marchesani's syndrome. Both of these entities have skeletal abnormalities and problems with the lens in the eye.

Marfan's syndrome often presents with increased length of the long bones in the arms and legs which makes the child tall and thin. The fingers and toes may be longer than usual for the child's age. These patients often have a high arched palate, stretched ligaments and may have congenital heart diseases and deformity of the spine.

The usual ocular problem is dislocation of the lens resulting is the lens only partially filling the pupil so that the child must look both around and through the edge of the lens. When looking through the part of the pupil that is not covered by the lens, the eye is very far sighted and must be corrected with the post cataract removal type of glasses or contact lens. With this correction the child often sees better than they can by looking through the edge of the dislocated lens. Both eyes must be treated the same way. The brain cannot fuse the image from an eye seeing through a human lens with the image from an eye seeing through post cataract glasses. The image through the post cataract glasses is thirty to forty percent larger than the normal image through the lens, so the brain cannot fuse it with normal sized image from the good eye. Contact lens fitting in infants and small children is very difficult, but possible

A child with Marfan's syndrome may also have high myopia, megalocornea, glaucoma and/or a cataract.

In Marchesani's syndrome, the child is often short and has fingers and toes that appear to be the same length, ending in a straight line. There is delayed ossification of the bones of the hands and feet.

The lens is dislocated and may be more rounded or spherical than normal causing the eye to become myopic (nearsighted).

This is associated with glaucoma, a common complication of dislocation of the lens from other causes.

There are many inborn errors of metabolism that affect the eye.

There are a number of enzymatic disorders that cause eye problems including errors of glycosaminoglycan metabolism (mucopolysaccharide metabolism if you took biochemistry before 1965).

They are grouped under the heading of gargoylism. The syndromes that affect the eye include Hurler's syndrome, (also known as Scheie's syndrome), Marquio's syndrome, and Maroteaux-Lamy syndrome. These eye problems may include megalocornea, glaucomatous ocular enlargement, pigmentary retinopathy, and optic atrophy. Hunter's syndrome does not involve the eye. Diagnosis and treatment of these various metabolic disorders requires a good endocrinologist and a good ophthalmologist.

Other metabolic diseases of childhood that involve the eye include cystinosis, homocystinuria, and galactosemia. These children are usually very sick from the systemic effects of the abnormal metabolism and the eye findings are incidental, sometimes aiding in the diagnosis.

Albinism is a hereditary defect in the metabolism of melanin.

It may be generalized or confined to the eyes. The iris is white to light blue, or pink in color, the retina is pale and the macula may not develop normally leaving the child with poor vision. This type of poor vision may lead to nystagmus of the searching type. Many people with albinism often develop a high degree of astigmatism, further complicating their visual problems.

When the albinism is generalized, the skin is pale, the hair, eyebrows and lashes are white, making the diagnosis readily apparent. When the hair and skin color are normal, the diagnosis is made of the appearance of the iris and retina. Albinism can be transmitted genetically by either the dominant, recessive, or sex linked patterns. A detailed history by a geneticist is necessary to determine the means and probability of passing the gene to offspring.

Several hereditary diseases of the eye involve the retina.

The most common of these is retinitis pigmentosa, often called RP. Retinitis pigmentosa is a group of hereditary diseases that involve the retinal receptor cells. Many gene mutations have been discovered that can cause RP. Because of the many mutations, the disease can be transmitted in autosomal dominant, autosomal recessive, or X-linked manner.

In the autosomal dominant transmission, one abnormal gene, from either the father or mother, will overpower the normal gene from the other parent. The recessive abnormal gene will be overpowered by the normal gene from the other parent, so matching genes from both parents must be abnormal. Both parents must be carriers of the abnormal gene. In the X-linked transmission, the abnormal gene is on the X, or female, gene from the mother.

When combined with a Y gene in a male, the X-linked gene will express itself. If it is combined with the X gene of the father who is normal, the girl will not express the disease. In X-linked transmission, women are carriers while boys are affected. In retinitis pigmentosa the X-linked gene can express in male offspring.

Clinically this disease presents as loss of peripheral vision and difficulty with night vision. The disease usually begins in the midperipheral retina. The rods degenerate, followed by degeneration of the surrounding retina and cones and the pigment epithelium.

The pigment migrates and clumps along the retinal vessels in a pattern that mimics bone spicules as seen under the microscope.

This pattern is very specific for this disease allowing its diagnosis.

Testing retinal function with the electroretinogram and the electro-oculogram may confirm the presence of the disease before it is clinically apparent. Electrical activity of the retina is markedly reduced in both of these tests.

The first symptom is usually night blindness. This may occur in the teen ages or early twenties. Progression is slow, but some patients lose almost all peripheral vision by the late twenties and early thirties. This progresses to tunnel vision in most patients by their forties or fifties. Some patients will then lose all central vision.

There are clinical and laboratory tests to confirm the diagnosis and determine which of the varieties of retinitis pigmentosa is present. These include color vision testing, fluorescein angiography, visual field testing, electroretinogram, electro-oculogram, and dark adaptation.

Genetic testing can be done on the patient and the parents to determine the probable course of the disease and the means and likelihood of transmission to future children. At least 35 different genes have been identified to be related to retinitis pigmentosa.

DNA testing is commonly available for nine specific gene changes. Testing for others may be available in research laboratories.

Genetic counseling depends on careful determination of the mode of inheritance, genetic testing and an accurate diagnosis.

RP can be associated with other diseases including deafness (Usher syndrome); obesity, mental retardation, hypogenitalism, and polydactyly (extra fingers or toes) (Laurence-Moon-Biedl syndrome); and several other very rare medical syndromes.

While there is no cure for retinitis pigmentosa, there are several treatments that help retard the progression. Vitamin A has been shown to retard the progression to blindness by as much as ten years. Vitamin A is available as a retinal implant. This means that the implant is placed in the eye to deliver vitamin A directly to the retina.

Research is being done with artificial (electronic) retinal implants, gene therapy, and stem cells, as well as nutritional and drug therapies. A company has just received permission to try a new therapy which involves medication mediated removal of a substance believed to cause retinitis pigmentosa.

There is one form of RP that does not show pigment changes in the retina. It is called retinitis pigmentosa sine pigmenti. It is diagnosed by visual symptoms and electrophysiological testing.

Two other inherited diseases affect the macula of the retina at an early age. Stargardt-Behr disease is transmitted in the dominant manner and causes macular pigment epithelium degeneration.

This leads to degeneration of the photoreceptor cells and loss of central vision. The degree of degeneration varies, but is similar within families.

Best's maculopathy is also autosomal dominant and occurs at an early age. Signs of the disease occur before vision is lost. A yellow deposit develops in the macula area within the pigment epithelium. It appears as an egg yolk in the macula. As the disease progresses, the yolk breaks and forms a scar in the macula that destroys central (reading) vision. There is no cure for either of these diseases, but genetic counseling is important as well as preparing these children for loss of central vision, i.e. learning Braille, learning to use peripheral vision and magnifiers.

INDEX

A

abducens nerve, 46, 49
accommodation, 276-80
accommodative convergence, 277, 280
accommodative esotropia, 278, 280
acquired immunodeficiency syndrome, 73, 203, 269-72,
acute angle closure glaucoma, 62, 175, 179, 192-4 189, 191
adenocarcinoma, 39
adenoviruses, 293
adult onset diabetes, 238
    far sighted shift in vision, 238
age related macular degeneration, 211-218
AIDS, 73, 198, 240-248
    fungal infections, 222, 247
    herpes infections, 245-8
    Kaposi sarcoma, 248
    opportunistic infections, 245-6
albinism 286, 299
allergic reactions, 7, 21, 42

Alport's syndrome, 271
alternate cover testing, 282
alternating esotropia, 280, 284
amblyopia, 251, 260-1, 268 271, 281-4
aneurysms, 9, 233, 245
angle closure glaucoma, 62, 175-7, 179, 182-4, 191
    peripheral iridectomy, 62, 163, 190, 192
anhidrosis, 257
aniridia, 196, 258, 266
ankylosing spondylitis, 34, 222,
anterior chamber, 28, 61, 128, 153, 158, 220
anterior segment necrosis, 290
anterior uveitis, 73
anti neovascular treatment, 216
anti VEGF, 96
anti VEGF drugs, 105, 219
ARMD, 211-218, 234
Amsler Grid, 214-5
ARED study, 215-6
    cures tried, 210

dry type, 211, 215
implantable telescope, 214
wet type, 210-4, 216-7
astigmatism, 51, 77, 112, 118, 146,, 209, 286, 300
atopic dermatitis, 196
Avastin, 219

B

basal cell carcinoma, 39-40
Behcet's disease, 73
Best's maculopathy, 302
bifocals, 77, 109, 114, 120
bimedial recession, 287
birth mark, 260
blepharitis, 15-9, 22, 24
    eye makeup, 19
    from chemotherapy, 16, 248, 270
    infectious, 24, 31
    seborrheic, 15, 24
blepharophimosis, 253, 259
blow out fracture, 56-9, 230
    double vision, 57
blue sclera, 272
brain tumors, 48, 50, 109, 223, 228
branch retinal artery occlusion, 92, 94
branch retinal vein occlusion, 95
burning eyes, 21

C

Candida, 66, 247, 294
capillary hemangioma, 260
    treatment, 261
capsule opacity, 123, 164
    in children, 267-8
capsulotomy, 165, 268-9
carcinoma in situ, 32
cataract, 130-65
    childhood, 268
    glare testing, 133
    posterior sub-capsular, 131
    removal timing, 133, 135
    symptoms, 132
    viral diseases, 267-8
cataract removal
    one eye or both, 133-5
cataract sugery, 138-165
    preparation, 141
cataract surgeon, 148-51
cataract complications, 151
    capsular opacity, 164
    contact lenses after, 145
    corneal edema, 157-9
    dislocated implant lens, 162-4
    dropped lens material, 160-2
    glasses after, 145-7
    infection, 155-7
    intraocular lenses, 127-9
    post-op restrictions, 141-3
    procedure, 138-41
    retinal detachment, 159-60
cavernous sinus disease, 227
CD 4 cells, 245
central areolar choroidal sclerosis, 218
central retinal artery occlusion, 4, 92-4, 96, 101, 246

glaucoma, 177, 234
   medication induced, 96
central retinal vein occlusion, 94-5
cerebellar tumors, 228
chalazion, 38-9
chemical injury, 11, 21, 24, 130
chicken pox, 48, 294
Chlamydia, 7, 9-10, 274, 294
choroid, 59, 154-5, 166, 186-9, 212, 218-9, 223, 246, 253, 267, 286
choroiditis, 73, 258
Chron's disease, 34, 222
chronic simple glaucoma, 4, 76, 173-5, 180, 191
ciliary body, 60-1, 141, 166, 172, 182, 219, 290
coccidiomycosis, 247
Cogan/Guerry dystrophy, 197
coloboma, 257, 266-7
color blindness, 98-101
color changes, 98-102, 144
comotio retinae, 58,
congenital eye defects, 258-62
congenital eye problems, 251
congenital glaucoma, 266-7
congenital orbital teratoma, 262-7
conjunctiva, 4 6, 13, 21, 30, 255
Conjunctivitis
   allergic, 7, 10, 19-21, 42 bacterial, 6-7, 14, 274
connective tissue diseases, 298
cornea, 28, 157-9, 196, 290
   thermal burn, 11, 198
edema, 28, 157-9,, 196, 267, 290

foreign body, 25-9, 71-2,
corneal dystrophies, 194, 198
corneal scarring, 199, 251-2
corneal transplant, 52, 152, 157-9, 193-210
   Eye Banks, 201-4
   procedure, 204
   sutures, 206, 208-9
corneal transplant types, 199
   deep anterior lamellar keratoplasty, 199
   disk of Descemet's membrane, 20
   layer of endothelial cells, 200
   penetrating keratoplasty, 64-5, 197-9
   post op restrictions, 207
corneal trasnsplants
   results, 209
corneal ulcers, 4, 11, 18,122, 198-200, 240
cover testing, 282
cranial nerve palsies, 45-50, 226
   treatment, 229
Credé prophylaxis, 273
crossed eyes, 45-52, 275-289
crystalline lens, 3, 258
curtains and shadows, 3-4, 59, 80-91
Cyclosporin A, 23, 30, 35, 201
cyst, eyelid, 38, 261
cystinosis, 299
cystoid macular edema CME, 135, 151-2
cytomegalovirus, 247

D

dacryocystorhinostomy, 257
Dalmane, 13
damage to central vision, 77, 84, 95, 301-2
depth perception, 49, 90, 134, 142, 224, 251-2, 281-5
dermoid, 266
dermoid tumors, 42, 261
diabetes, 232-9
    cataract formation, 237
    central retinal artery occlusion, 234
    central retinal vein occlusion, 234
    fourth cranial nerve palsy, 233
    neovascularization of the iris, 237
    new vessels on the retina, 235
    sixth cranial nerve palsy, 233
    third cranial nerve palsy, 233
diabetes and the eye, 232-39
    underlying cause, 232
diabetic retinopathy, 234
    lazers in, 122, 235
digitalis, 100
diplopia, 51, 229
direct laser photocoagulation, 216
double vision, 3, 45-52, 120, 226-31, 240-3, 282-3
Down's syndrome, 65, 196
dry eyes, 22-3, 33-6, 74, 240, 257
    burning sensation, 21
    medication related, 17, 35
    treatment, 35
Duane's syndrome, 229

E

Ehlers Danlos syndrome, 272
embryology, 251-4
encephalitis, 246, 252
endophthalmitis, 65, 155-6
    metastatic, 65
    pain, 156
    vitrectomy, 157
epicanthus., 257
epikeratophakia, 126-7
epilepsy, 296
epiretinal membrane, 170
    vitrectomy and peeling, 171
esotropia, 275-82
    accomodative, 178, 280
    alternating, 280, 284
exotropia, 275-83
expulsive hemorrhage, 154-5
extraocular muscles, 8, 226-31, 241, 253
eye injury, 58
eye lashes,, 17, 19, 30, 40, 183
eye problems of children, 40, 42, 45, 53, 107, 164, 178, 204, 249-302
eye rubbing, 21, 25, 87
eye socket, 13, 32, 42,, 56-8, 229-31, 243, 261
eye straightening surgery, 288
eyebrows, 300

eyelids, 10-12, 15-7, 38-40, 53-5,2240, 259
Eylea, 217

F

familial dysautonomia, 257
    Riley Day syndrome, 257
familial shallow orbit syndrome, 43
Fasanella procedure, 260
flare and cells, 220
flashes and floaters, 80-91, 160, 168
    fireworks, 80, 160, 167
    lightning streaks, 81
flax seed, 26
floaters, 81-91
forceps delivery, 267
foreign bodies, 25-7
fourth cranial nerve (CN IV) palsy, 46, 48. 228
    children with cerebellar tumors, 228
    frontal blow to the head, 228
fourth nerve palsy, 48, 228
Fuch's dystrophy, 158-9, 195, 199
fungus, 66, 195, 294

G

galactosemia, 299
gargoylism, 3299
gill pouches, 259
glaucoma, 60, 172-92,
    acute, 60, 177
    children, 179, 267
    chronic simple, 4, 76, 172-4, 180, 188, 191
    computerized cameras, 182
    congenital, 266-7
    dislocated lens, 299
    eye drops, 182
    FDA drug labeling, 191
    juvenile, 178-9
    malignant, 62
    optic nerve in, 76-7, 173-5
    peripheral iridectomy, 61, 163, 190, 192
    plateau iris, 62-3
    pupillary block, 175
    sneak theif of vision, 5,, 175
    traumatic, 179
    treatment, 180
glaucoma surgery, 184
    cyclo-cryo therapy, 187-8
    cyclodialysis, 185-7
    setons, rods and tubes, 187
    trabeculectomy, 185
glaucoma treatment
    lasers, 184
    medications, 61, 180, 182-4
glycosaminoglycan, 8-9, 241, 299
gonorrhea, 247, 273
Grave's eye disease, 240

H

halos around lights, 175
hazy cornea, 28, 35, 153, 175, 179, 267
head trauma, 13, 74, 96
head turning, 285-6, 291

headache, 3, 50, 63, 73, 77-9, 87, 96
    ophthalmic migraine, 79-80
Hemophilus Egyptius, 293
hereditary diseases in children, 298-302
herpes simplex, 4, 8, 27-9, 49, 221-3, 246
    disciform keratitis, 28
    oral antivirals, 29, 247
    steroids, 28
herpes zoster, 49, 246
    shingles, 48, 246
heterochromia of the iris, 219
high blood pressure, 45-8, 92, 96, 112, 215, 246
histoplasmosis, 73, 247
HIV, 245-8
    cotton wool spots, 245-7
    Hemorrhages, 245-6
    telangiectasia, 245
    vascular aneurysms, 245
HLA B27, 245-8
homocystinuria, 299
hordeolum, 37
Horner's syndrome, 54, 219
human immunodeficiency virus, 245
Hurler's syndrome, 299
hydroxychloroquine (Plaquinil), 96, 101
hypermature cataract, 131, 155
hyperopia, 104, 111-2, 121, 125
hypertension, 45-8, 92, 96, 112, 215, 246
hyperthyroid disease, 240-2

hyphema, post op, 152
hypothyroid disease, 42, 242

I

inferior oblique muscle, 46-8, 226, 229, 232, 285
infrared light, 144-45
intracranial aneurysm, 47
intraocular lenses, 18, 62, 68, 117, 126-9,, 142-7
    in children, 179
    myopia, 129
    new designs, 147
intraocular membrane, 58
iris, 40, 60-3, 65, 128, 175, 189, 219-22, 237, 258, 266-9, 286, 290, 300
    color, 219
iritis, 73, 220
itchy burning eyes, 21-4

K

Kaposi Sarcoma, 248
keratoconus, 51-2, 64
    hydrops, 64-5
keratoprostheses, 198
kidney disease, 42, 221, 233

L

lacrimal canaliculi, 23, 36, 255-7
lacrimal duct obstruction, 256
    spontaneous opening, 256
lacrimal glands, 256

lacrimal problems, 255-7
lacrimal sac, 255
Lasik, 124
lazy eye, 251, 260-1, 281-4
lenticonus, 271
leprosy, 40
leukemia, 73, 222
leukemia and lymphoma, 222
levator muscle, 746, 54, 227, 259-60
Librium, 13, 35, 191-2
lice, 17
lid lag, 240-1
lid retraction, 240
low tension glaucoma, 174
Lucentis, 217
lumps and bumps, 38-41

M

Macugen, 217
macular degeneration, 211-7
    symptoms, 213
Marchesani's syndrome, 271-2, 298-9
Marfan's syndrome, 271-2
Maroteaux-Lamy syndrome, 299
Marquio's syndrome, 299
Masquerade syndrome, 223
measles, 48-9, 73, 252, 258, 267, 294
megalocornea, 266, 272, 294
melanoma, 40, 225
meningeal irritation, 73-4
meningioma, 42, 227
meningitis, 49, 73, 228, 246
metabolic malfunction, 298
micro cornea, 266-7

microphthalmus, 258, 266
mid facial syndrome, 253-4
migraine, 48, 73
miosis, 277
Molluscum contagiosum, 40
monocular diplopia, 51
mono fit lenses, 117
multiple sclerosis, 48
mumps, 294
muscle palsies, 226-31, 233
myasthenia gravis, 48, 53, 229
myopia, 48, 53, 105-20, 121-30, 132, 167, 178, 196,, 228, 251, 281, 299

N

nasolacrimal duct, 255-6
    probing, 256
necrotizing scleromalacia, 225
neonatal ophthalmia, 273
neurofibroma, 40
neurofibromatosis, 40-2
NO SPECS, 242
NVD, 234
NVE, 235
nystagmus, 291, 300
    congenital jerk, 291
    null point, 291
    searching, 291

O

oblique muscles, 45-8,, 226, 233, 285-9

occipital cortex, 295
ocular cicatricial pemphigoid, 30, 198, 203
ocular enlargement, 198
ocular prolapse, 44
oculomotor nerve, 46, 259
optic atrophy, 246, 294, 299
optic nerve, 42, 44, 76-7, 80-2, 92-3, 96, 109, 154, 173-84, 228, 234, 241-3, 2246, 251, 267, 295
optic nerve contusion, 96-7
optic nerve glioma, 42
optic nerve transection, 96-7
optical confusion, 285
oral glaucoma treatment, 184
    Diamox, 184
orbit, 42-3, 56-8, 230, 242-4, 261-6
osteogenesis imperfecta, 272

P

pain, 60-79
    at 2 am, 92, 154
    dull aching, 60, 65, 72
    glaucoma, 4, 60, 163, 175
    hard contact lenses, 64
    on awakening, 12
persistant foreign body, 27, 70
papilledema, 93, 96,228
parasites, 73, 221, 294
parasitic worm, 297
pars planitis, 73
patching, 64, 271, 282-5
periarteritis nodosa, 73

permanent eye liner, 20
phacoemulsification, 140, 150
phoria, 274-5, 282, 285
photo dynamic therapy (PDT), 216
photo refractive keratectomy (PRK), 124
photophobia, 73-4, 220
pigmentary retinopathy, 299
pinguecula, 32-3
pink eye, 7, 9, 219, 293-4
Plaquinil, 96, 101
pneumococcus, 293
pollens, 21, 294
polycoria, 267
polyneuritis, 49
post operative hyphema, 153
posterior scleritis, 224-5
presbyopia, 77, 111, 114, 117
progressive lenses, 115-9
prominent eyes, 43, 240
proptosis, 240-2
pseudotumor cerebrii, 50, 96, 228
pseudoxanthoma elasticum, 272
psoriasis, 222
pterygium, 31
ptosis, 53-5
    treatment, 53
pupil, 54, 58, 61-3, 131-2, 163, 172, 177, 219-21, 227, 233, 237, 260-1, 267-70, 376-7, 296-7

R

radial keratotomy, 122-3
rapid vision loss, 92

reading glasses, 117-9, 130 147,
    drug store readers, 118
recess and resect, 287-8
rectus muscles, 455-6, 226, 230-3, 287, 290
recurrent erosions, 12-3, 197-8
    treatment, 13
red eye, 3-4, 6-14, 26, 32, 175, 294
    noninfectious, 10, 11-3
red out eye drops, 14
red rimmed eyes, 15
refractive disorders, 105-120
reticulum cell sarcoma, 73
retina, 4, 56-9, 80-91, 92-6, 101, 135, 159-62, 166-71, 211-7, 218-74, 296-7, 299
retina holes, 83, 160
retinal damage, 258
retinal detachment, 82.5, 111, 142, 151-2, 159-62, 166-71, 268-71
    massage vibrators, 167
    myopia, 167
    scleral buckle, 169
    symptoms, 167
    treatment, 168-70
retinitis pigmentosa, 196, 300
    sine pigmenti, 302
retinoblastoma, 269-70
retinopathy of prematurity, 269
retrolental fibroplasias, 269
rhabdomyosaroma, 42, 263-6
rheumatoid arthritis, 23, 34
rheumatoid diseases, 12, 73, 34, 72, 127, 222-4

rickettsia, 294
Rocky Mountain spotted fever, 294
RP, 196, 300-2
Rubella, 258, 267, 294

S

sarcoidosis, 73, 220-1
sebaceous cyst, 261
second cataract removal, 135
secondary deviations, 284
seizure, 295-6
senile keratosis, 40
severe dry eye disease, 35, 198
shingles, 48, 246
signs, 3
silver nitrate, 273-4
sinusitis, 49
sixth cranial nerve, 46, 50, 228, 233
sixth cranial nerve (CN VI) palsy, 49, 228
    pseudotumor, 50, 96, 228
sixth nerve palsy, 49, 226
Sjögren's syndrome, 23, 34-5
    treatment, 34-5
Sjögren's Syndrome Foundation, 35
skin cancers, 39-40
squamous cell carcinoma, 39
staphylococcus, 67, 274, 294
Stargardt Behr disease, 302
status epilepticus, 296
stereoscopic vision, 284
Stevens Johnson syndrome, 17-9, 198, 203
strabismus, 45, 274

strabismus surgery, 281, 287-90
    procedure, 288
strange eyelid movements, 240
streptococcus, 294
stress, 27, 77, 252
stroke, 45-50, 109
sty, 38
sub retinal membrane, 170
sulfacetamide, 274
superior oblique muscle, 48, 226, 233, 285, 295
suppression of the brain, 283-4
synkinetic near response, 277, 280
syphilis, 73, 203, 247, 273
systemic lupus erythematosus, 34, 40

T

T cells, 245
tearing, 7, 33, 255-7
tears, 22, 33-4, 255-7,
    components, 22
    hypotonic artificial, 23
telecanthus, 253, 259
tendon sheath tenotomy, 289
teratoma, 261, 262-6
testing ocular alignment, 282
tetracycline, 10, 16-7, 50, 76, 274
third cranial nerve, 46-7, 233
third cranial nerve palsy, 46, 55, 226, 233,
    pupil responses, 49, 227
thyroid disease, 42, 240-4
thyroid eye disease, 45, 240-4
    orbital decompression, 243

strabimus surgery, 243
    treatment, 242-3
TIA, transcient ischemic attack, 95
toxocariasis, 221, 269
toxoplasmosis, 73, 220, 246-7, 258, 294
trabecular meshwork, 62, 173-5, 177-8
Trachoma, 31, 294
trauma, 13, 45-9, 57, 73, 89, 96, 130, 166, 179-80, 193, 196, 223, 227-30, 247, 267
trichiasis, 31
Trichinella, 294
trifocals, 114, 126-7
trisomy 65
trochlear nerve, 46, 48
tropia, 274-5, 282-3
tuberculosis, 7, 73, 200-2, 241

U

ulcerative colitis, 222
ultraviolet light, 11, 27, 144, 162-4, 235
uveitis, 32, 40, 65, 73, 219-25
    granulomatous, 220
    non-granulomatous, 222
    treatment, 221-4

V

Valium, 13, 35,191-2
vascular endothelial growth factor, 95-112, 217, 234

VEGF, 195, 212, 217, 235, 245
vernal keratitis, 29
Viagra, 96, 100
viral conjunctivitis, 6-9, 294
viral diseases, 7-8, 48, 222, 258, 268, 294
vision change, 4, 100
vision without glasses, 121-9, 144-5,
visual field testing, 109, 185, 301
Visudyne, 216
vitamin A, 12, 50, 198, 301-2
vitamin A deficiency, 12, 50, 198, 301-2
vitrectomy, 59, 85, 89-90, 161-2, 169, 236,
vitreous, 58, 62. 73, , 80-2, 135, 152, 1156-7, 167
vitreous hemorrhages, 58, 86, 88-9, 101, 236
    diabetic, 88-9, 236
vitreous membranes, 88, 108, 236
Vosious' Ring, 221

W

wall eyes, 45, 252
welder's burn, 11, 64
wet ARMD, 211-2, 216-7
    modern treatments, 214-5, 216-7
white pupil, 267-9, 286-7

Y

YAG laser, 68, 165, 190, 269

Z

zonular cataract, 258, 268

www.ingramcontent.com/pod-product-compliance
Lightning Source LLC
Chambersburg PA
CBHW020726180526
45163CB00001B/127